PENGUIN

MADNESS
a memoir

Kate Richards is a writer of narrative non-fiction, fiction and poetry. She holds a medical degree with honours from Monash University and a diploma of arts from RMIT University, where she won the 2012 Judy Duffy Prize for literary excellence. She works in medical research.

MADNESS

a memoir

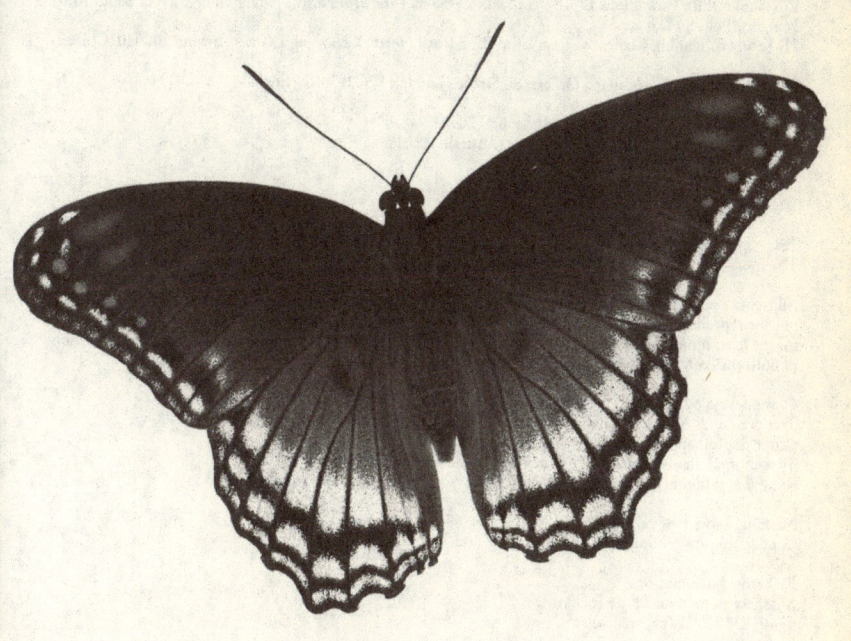

KATE RICHARDS

PENGUIN BOOKS

PENGUIN

Published by the Penguin Group
Penguin Group (Australia)
707 Collins Street, Melbourne, Victoria 3008, Australia
(a division of Penguin Australia Pty Ltd)
Penguin Group (USA) Inc.
375 Hudson Street, New York, New York 10014, USA
Penguin Group (Canada)
90 Eglinton Avenue East, Suite 700, Toronto, Canada ON M4P 2Y3
(a division of Penguin Canada Books Inc.)
Penguin Books Ltd
80 Strand, London WC2R 0RL England
Penguin Ireland
25 St Stephen's Green, Dublin 2, Ireland
(a division of Penguin Books Ltd)
Penguin Books India Pvt Ltd
11 Community Centre, Panchsheel Park, New Delhi – 110 017, India
Penguin Group (NZ)
67 Apollo Drive, Rosedale, Auckland 0632, New Zealand
(a division of Penguin New Zealand Pty Ltd)
Penguin Books (South Africa) (Pty) Ltd
Rosebank Office Park, Block D, 181 Jan Smuts Avenue, Parktown North, Johannesburg, 2196, South Africa
Penguin (Beijing) Ltd
7F, Tower B, Jiaming Center, 27 East Third Ring Road North, Chaoyang District, Beijing 100020, China

Penguin Books Ltd, Registered Offices: 80 Strand, London WC2R 0RL, England

First published by Penguin Group (Australia), 2013
This edition published by Penguin Group (Australia), 2014

10 9 8 7 6 5 4 3 2 1

Text copyright © Kate Richrads, 2013
The moral right of the author has been asserted

Cover design by Alex Ross © Penguin Group (Australia)
Text design by Allison Colpoys © Penguin Group (Australia)
Cover photograph © Valentino Sani/Trevillion Images
Typeset in Garamond by Post Pre-press Group, Brisbane, Queensland
Printed and bound in Australia by McPherson's Printing Group, Maryborough, Victoria

National Library of Australia
Cataloguing-in-Publication data:

Richards, Kate, author.
Madness : a memoir / Kate Richards.
9780143571391 (paperback)
Richards, Kate.
Psychoses–Patients–Biography.
Women physicians–Biography.

616.890092

penguin.com.au

Madness is a real world for the many thousands of people who are right now living within it and dying within it. It never apologises. Sometimes it is a shadow, ever present, without regard for the sun. Sometimes it is a well of dark water with no bottom, or a levitation device to the stars. It takes away the rational minds of ordinary people. It takes our hearts, knowing death so well. This world was once my pair of horns, my pair of wings. Now we regard each other with caution and, yes, healthy respect. Both bruised but very much alive.

This book is for everyone living within this world, for everyone touched by this world, and for everyone seeking to further his or her understanding of it, whether you think of madness as a biological illness of the brain or an understandable part of the continuum of the human condition. Either way, we – the people who inhabit this world – are in every other respect just like you. We want to live well.

This memoir relies on the many volumes of notes, observations, conversations, odd phrases and sudden ideas written during episodes of illness and transcribed here unedited. It also relies on memory, which is commonly subjective and fragile, and on the notes of treating clinicians. The events took place over a period of about fifteen years. In the interests of telling a story, time is on occasion expanded and on occasion compressed.

The names of individuals (and in some cases their gender and physical appearance) have been altered to preserve anonymity except where permission has been granted.

1

Flirting. With burning, injecting, infection, ash, caustic soda and perfume. Eyes, dry and hot, lie heavy in their bony sockets. I am going to cut off my right arm. This is an operation like any other, with the exception of anaesthesia. I have procured a surgeon's scalpel, a stitch cutter, a chef's knife, surgical scissors, tweezers, needle and syringe.

A third of the way down from my shoulder to elbow the scalpel slides over and into my white skin, dimly freckled and smooth as mango. Skin is surprisingly recalcitrant. The part of my mind that is consciousness has folded itself away. I am blank. The scalpel finds the deepest skin, the dermis, the little yellow pillows of fat like pearls. Bluish-red bloodlines seep down my right arm, over my right breast.

It is true that blood is thicker than water. Blood doesn't run in the way of water. It is glutinous, it has a richness. As a symbol, is inextricably linked to the colour red. It lies at the end of a series that begins with sunlight and yellow-gold. It is the perfect symbol of animate life, of passion, of sacrifice.

Getting up, I go and look at the arm in the mirror, I breathe awkwardly; my heartbeat is awkward in my ears. The sky in the mirror is grey with patchy clouds and a low red sun. My cat sits on the bed impassively. I breathe in more than air. There is an exquisite burning, prickling pain in my head and down the right side of my body. The stitch cutter is useful for usurping bits of fibrous connective tissue that bind the body together. I cut deeper and widen the wound with the surgical scissors. Blood is running thickly, clotting in warm lumps along my arm, inching along cracks in the floorboards.

My hands are both shaking so I enclose the bad hand in the good hand for a moment, hold them, then press the scalpel in deeper. The wind has picked up, it is quite dark, the corners of the room are looming into the wider space with their quiet cream plaster, everything is suddenly round and small and I am breathing low, long breaths with a kind of rasp at the end – more than a sigh, less than a wail. This is a private relationship – me and the air and the room and the scalpel in my hands, the blood at my feet. But I can't get further than the pure blue-white of bone – there is too much red, the smell of acetic acid and warmed metal, the redundant tissue, and my fingers have gone quite cold. I leave the instruments on the floor and wrap up my arm in a blue bath towel. The other people who live in my head – the ones who bicker and sneer and cajole and scream – they are at last still. Atonement, I think, appeasement. A little death.

It is 3 a.m. the morning after. Outside the local hospital the wind is brisk and the lights fluorescent. Cars whip by; flashes in the night. The Emergency Department waiting room is small; a sign above the main desk says Triage Nurse. I sit down and wait. A young man arrives behind the desk, sits, looks at the chart in front of him, makes a phone call, taps into the computer. Then he says, 'Can I help you?'

'I tried to cut off my arm.'

'Pardon?'

'My arm . . .' Blood is a blush through my shirt.

'How did this happen?'

'I tried to cut it off.'

'When?'

'Last night.'

'Oh.' Then, 'Why did you wait so long to come in?' I shrug my one good shoulder and stare at the linoleum floor.

The triage area looks out across the road and the tram tracks to a large park, whose closest trees are lit yellow-white by the hospital lights. The sky backs black and voluminous. My head has left my body and is floating somewhere just below a corner of the roof.

Deeper inside the Emergency Department the smell is a mixture of urine and bleach and something I can't define. I take my clothes off and am left alone in a white cotton gown. The cubicle has pink curtains. I doze briefly. People are paged, IV pumps bleep, the air ambulance phone rings into the night. I lie and think and poke at my thick hot arm. The Plastics Registrar, a small man with slick black hair and pinstriped pants, decides on surgery. 'Now,' he says, white coat tails disappearing down the white corridor. He has left the towels in a darkly red pile in the corner of the room. My arm leers open, a hopeless mix of skin, muscle fibre and the pearlescent globs of fat. Blood seeps thickly.

The anaesthetics registrar is kind. She takes my good hand and smiles. I'm flooded with something like relief and then confusion. After surgery I wake in a hospital bed with my arm strapped down at my side. An IV line runs delicately from my other arm into a bag of normal saline above my head. It is connected to a blue pump that has flashing yellow numbers on its front and bleeps and whines periodically; it is talking. The curtains are open and outside the dark is not black, rather a dull orange brown. It is cool and quiet and ordered and I feel like oozing through the bed and the floor and out into the night.

'Patient Controlled Analgesia,' says the nurse, patting an electronic pad on my left. 'Morphine.' I press the button. There is a whoosh along my veins from finger tips to heart, which flutters, I have several orgasms, I'm as relaxed as it is possible to be, suddenly the sky above is very blue – there are no clouds.

Later a surgical resident stands at the end of the bed in a perfect blue suit, a continuation of the sky. 'We've sewn up the biceps muscle belly and the triceps tendons. You missed the brachial artery; otherwise you probably wouldn't be here. The plaster cast needs to stay on for four weeks to let everything heal. We won't know whether you've lost any function until we take it off. Exercising your fingers is fine.'

I sit up. There appears to be a camera in the overhead light and another one in the air conditioning vent. This is some kind of test. My fingers are bright orange from the iodine pre-surgical wash. They aren't connected to me at all. The rest of my arm up to the shoulder is immobilised by a plaster cast curved at the elbow and covered with a bandage and tape. I can't go to the toilet with the cameras in the room and the pain from my bladder radiates.

This killing is a killing of part of the self. Removing an arm, removing a symbolic tumour, severing something unnatural. I know. I know how to get the rotten bits out, under the stone-eyed stare of the people in my head. They are a little like God. Greater. Stronger. Wiser.

Two security guards flank the wheelchair while a nurse from the surgical ward wheels me along the shiny linoleum from the main hospital to Psychiatry. There is no caffeine in the High Dependency Unit. Cigarettes are regulated, lighters not allowed. HDU is five rooms locked off from the rest of the ward. My shoelaces, belt, toothbrush, shampoo, razor, tweezers, pens and deodorant have been taken away. Later they take my glasses. All of my senses are in chaos. I am a firefly without luciferase: instead of luminescence there is a dark that is engulfing and at the same time vacuous. I cannot see more than half a metre in front of my face; after that there is a joyous amalgam of colour and some vague suggestion of form.

No, I'm okay, I can't breathe. I ask staff to let me sleep in the main room where I can see other people. They refuse. I ask for more Largactil. They bring me 100 mg, which I take with a swig of fake coffee. I can't cry, but there is a howl lurking somewhere between my stomach and my diaphragm. The stitched up right arm throbs dully in its casing.

After the morning staff meeting the psych registrar calls me into an interview room where I meet the consultant psychiatrist and Lisa B, my contact nurse. The consultant conducts the interview, the registrar takes notes in a corner, Lisa sits next to me on the couch.

'How are you?' asks the consultant. I curl up, knees under my chin, then hold my hands out, palms upward and shrug. My hands shake. 'How are you,' is too enormous a question, there are too many possibilities, it is too vast a chasm to cross.

'How do you feel about being here?'

'Confused.'

'Why?'

'I should be dead.' The registrar writes that down.

'Why should you be dead, Kate?'

'It is the process of natural selection, it's in my DNA. I was born wrong.' No one appears to understand.

At lunch, beef stroganoff, carrots and beans, I meet a fellow patient with multicoloured layers of cloth winding up his wrists to his biceps and CARPE DIEM tattooed around the base of his neck in red and black. He smiles with his eyes as well as his mouth.

'I feel like jumping out of my skin every day of the week,' he says. His smile is infectious and his t-shirt reads 'Kill Your TV'.

'I'm not so flamboyant anymore. Now that I've got my head together, because before I used to be the prime minister you know but I had to resign. Are you smart? I am, but I have to be careful because it's likely that if they find out they'll be on to me, know what I mean? Bottom line is, I'm in disguise.'

I'm watching everyone from behind a glass wall, I am walking through treacle. Staff restrict my visitors until I take a shower. I can't see the point. They'll insist I do it all over again tomorrow.

Not even sleep is safe. This particular night a man is standing at the end of my bed with a knife. He has tied me on my back with scratchy white rope. He stands quite still in the dark. I can tell when he is blinking; I can see his sclerae. Cloth of some kind is forced down my throat. I stop breathing. There is flint and fumes and spirals of fluff in my throat, someone is caressing my neck. I stop breathing.

Usually I drown the dreams with wine, vodka, bourbon, anything. When alcohol is not enough, I add benzos: temazepam, mogadon, rivotril, and when they don't work, I throw in analgesics: codeine, doxylamine, tramadol, and finish up with the antihistamines: phenergan, chlorpheniramine. I lie in an absurd stupor for hours, but the dreams become smaller – flashes of violence in the night – a tight, concrete stairwell, a push in the small of the back, the falling, black and grey. At 3 a.m. my mouth is wide-open, tongue dry as sand, hands in fists.

Someone is pacing and angry. Someone else is out cold on the floor. Staff wake him up and march him to his room. He's shuffling terribly. I watch from the corner, my back to the cool walls.

There's a flash of colour across my eyes, a fist.

There's movement and shouting inside my head.

I sit absolutely still; I don't blink. Later I go into my cubicle and pull a long black sock out of a drawer and lie down on the prickly carpet that has a large stain in the centre and tie the sock around my neck with the ends facing front and I pull down hard on the ends and my ears are suddenly full of white noise, I'm sweating, I feel very light like I'm swaying in a easy breeze, I pull down harder and my head is quiet, I am suddenly tender, I wonder if I'm smiling, there is a Code Blue being called somewhere – somewhere someone's heart has stopped beating in between the cold and the air and the stretch of consciousness called reason.

2

The sun stirs on my face, its warmth slides across the divide in my head: a connection. I am out of seclusion, having been locked in for two days and two nights in a white gown in a white room with no socks. The white fluorescent light has mottled my skin and the people in my head are quiet. Staff have given back my glasses. The world is at once closer, sharper, more insistent, and with a combination of venlafaxine and lithium and diazepam it opens up even further, but with fewer teeth. I breathe, there are muted voices inside and outside, there is sunshine, cool wind, and I notice the way the leaves on the trees in the courtyard move in the wind.

The main ward is vinyl and concrete and perspex windows looking out onto the courtyard. Grey vinyl chairs, grey carpet, equally grey walls. Staff are kept safe from patients in a glass room in the centre of the unit, backing onto HDU. There is a television and a broken exercise bike and a broken rocking chair and an art room with a radio.

My mum and dad visit. Because the door to the ward is locked, they have to ring a bell and wait to be admitted by a member of staff. I'm on one side of the glass door, waiting, and they are on the other – the outside-world-side of the door, the normal side.

We don't talk much. We sit on the bed, me in the middle, and hold hands and their hands are strong and warm and they hold me for a moment together.

Later Hana and I drink coffee. Hana is a spoken word poet and musician, with a magnificent sense of rhythm. Her friends have brought in her guitar. She plays Elliott Smith . . . picking every note perfectly.

I take out one of my scruffy notebooks and write.

Rachel, one of the other women on the ward, gives us a foot spa in an old blue paint bucket. The smell of sandalwood and jasmine is finished off with lime; the warm oil-infused water feels like silk. I look at my naked legs in the water. The scars on my legs are pink and dark red and blue-grey – new skin, a fragile sleeve of skin that has crept over the little stories, little souls, little griefs that populate my insides.

My skin is too pure a cover for what lies underneath; I can't bear touch. There is something about the pureness of touch – skin to skin – that is intolerable. I shrink, flinch, cower, forget to breathe. Touch is a tiny request for opening up, for presenting one's underside for a shared second. Instead my hands do a kind of dance away from each other; there is a gap in my consciousness and I fall through it.

'I'm going home today,' Rachel says. I raise my eyebrows. Rachel still looks wild. She's thirty-one. This is her fifteenth hospitalisation. Her long brown hair is platted with strips of purple cotton and piled up in a bun on top of her head.

'Thank God. I want to go to New York.'

'Oh, yeah, me too,' says Hana. We laugh.

'Have you met my daughter?' Rachel asks.

'Not yet,' I reply.

Sky so blue today, if I were to
grasp it → black (how is it that
the earth spins and we do
not know?) ~~NO DAYLIGHT~~, furry eyesight
~~insight~~ so

in the night the mind opens
wide like a mouthful
of ~~teeth~~ a complete set of
~~my~~ incisors that ~~scissor swallow~~
seize the air and grind down
darkness.

~~'Belief' has loosened its chains~~ Register
all colour blood red. Conjure
bodies mountainous as ogres
~~three dimensional~~ shadows.
found blind —
                        foggy
blind between psyche + memory
Free nerves. **Free nerves.**

Leave the ends to reverberate
over — Daliesque visions that
melt and mould (mould) to the
gums on waking like stale milk.

without sense. How pain is.

'It's her birthday tomorrow.' She pauses. 'She's the most beautiful thing in the world. The most beautiful.' We nod.

'I would be dead without her. D'you know?'

We nod. Rachel's eyes grow luminous in the fluorescent overhead light.

She stands up suddenly, walks over to a man in a long black leather coat with hair reaching far out from the sides of his face and head. Rachel kisses him and runs her hands lightly down his cheeks. He smiles at her, all encompassing. I look away.

Staff give me a battery of neurocognitive tests on computer: attention, immediate recall, short-term memory, concentration, learning and executive function. I tap my head and shake it side to side like a dog, twist my scarf around my good hand, the pale blue chenille soft against my skin. My right arm lies heavy in its sling, the skin under the plaster itches, the fingers like worms move without purpose. Press the yes key when the card displayed is red.

Though the door is shut people periodically walk in. An elderly lady, who won't give her name, sits down on the floor in the corner and dozes off.

'What does all that glitters is not gold mean?' asks the registrar.

'Surface beauty doesn't equal inner substance,' I reply.

'Mmm,' he says. 'What about a fish out of water?'

'Unnatural situation.'

'And how are you today?'

'Okay.'

'Your bloods are good.'

'Terrific. Am I cured then?'

'Do you still want to die?'

'I still want to die.'

He walks away, I walk away.

Lisa B takes us for a walk under the trees in the park. Moving with anything like a purpose feels odd. We are bats suddenly blinded by light, we are awkward in the open space, unsure of the intent of our feet, except one young man, who takes off with the wind, running across the spiky grass in his big army boots, his arms stretched out toward the horizon either side of the sky.

Lisa B calls to him.

'Fuck off!' he shouts. He's tall and young and strong and he covers the ground at speed. Now Lisa's running too, lightly and fast, while the rest of us stand in an uncertain gaggle, bemused, shivering in spite of the sun.

Linda is my second roommate.

'Have you got a cigarette?' she asks, and gives me a toothless smile.

'No,' I say. 'Sorry.'

'Can I have your jumper then?'

'Um . . . no.' I say. 'Sorry. I've got some coffee, if you'd like.'

'Are you married?' she asks.

'No.'

'I am. Yesterday I was going to marry Peter, but today I'm in love with Darren.' She takes the coffee in a paper cup and disappears up the corridor. Later I return to our room to find all my clothes missing from the wardrobe. I sigh.

'I've washed them,' Linda says. Lying on the shower floor are indeed all my clothes – bras, knickers, socks, jeans– in a sodden, soapy pile. I'm back to the orange hospital pyjamas.

'Darren's taking me out tonight,' Linda says, sitting on my bed. 'We're gonna do it, you know . . . sex . . . there's this aura above us, sparkling, that's why it's gonna be tonight.' She starts to cry. I move over to her, almost touching her, we sit in the silence, quite still. She sniffs, 'I need him.' Linda leaves the curtain open while she undresses. Her belly is round as a cantaloupe and the skin of her torso and limbs is crazed, dusky pink as though minute rivers have eroded away its softness. Immolation?

I work with the ward psychologist on the tenets of cognitive-behavioural therapy: cognitions, assumptions, beliefs and behaviours. We discuss body image, I tell her my theory of the floating consciousness – freed from the body, free to inhabit the expanse of the universe much as a gas expands into the entire space in which it finds itself. She looks faintly troubled. Her hair is shining, it matches her eyes.

'There are some blank spaces,' I tell her, 'in my head.'

'Close your eyes,' she says. 'Concentrate on your breathing. Feel your feet on the floor. Now feel your calves, your thighs as they touch the seat. Your stomach, your back, your neck, your arms and hands, your fingers.' Her voice is soft. In the quiet the world reaches in from the outside. There is space around her words, for a moment I feel whole.

Then I meet a new patient at breakfast.

'All the usual suspects,' he says.

'Yes?'

'That was a rhetorical statement, bitch.'

I look up at him. 'Oh.' I say, confused.

'Listen,' he grabs my hair and leans into my face. 'I'm going to get my shotgun and shove it up your arse.' He says it very quietly, very intently.

I believe him.

'Keep away from me,' he hisses, letting me go.

I walk outside. Linda is talking on her mobile. She's wearing a long skirt, black and red, shimmery. On top she has a super tight skivvy to show off her belly. Rachel is talking with people from the

Mental Health Review Board. 'No, I'm completely cured,' she says. 'Actually, I was never sick in the first place, just overwrought.'

'Do you think the medication helps?'

'It makes me dopey. I can't think straight. I friggn' keep falling asleep!'

'Are you going to take it when you go home?'

'No way. Like I said, I can't keep my eyes open. I have to look after my daughter. I can't do that if I'm half asleep all day.' They nod up and down in unison and take copious notes.

Hana comes at me with a mouth full of chocolate. 'Kiss me,' she says. I kiss her. Her lips are soft as clouds. Simon laughs and makes a whooping noise; I punch him lightly in the ribs.

'That good?' he asks. 'Wish it were me.'

The ward courtyard has a garden containing a miniature Japanese maple with a curved trunk and several flowering gum trees. There's also a gnarled plane tree bereft of its leaves, the lower branches having been sawn off to prevent people climbing it. We sit in a circle by its trunk, drinking de-caffeinated coffee, watching the light change light grey to dark as the sun moves across the sky. I can't always make out who is talking.

Two weeks after admission, the unit social worker helps me complete forms to claim Sickness Allowance: $453.30 a fortnight. I can't tell if this is a lot of money or a pittance, the numbers sit unprocessed in my brain. And I have an appointment with the Plastic Surgery people. They remove the plaster cast on my arm with an electric saw. The stitches are ready to come out – a cut above the knot, a soft pull through skin – the wavery black string lying innocuous on stainless steel once held me together.

'ECT,' says the psychiatrist one morning. 'Electroconvulsive therapy.' She accentuates convulsive.

'Fabulous,' I say. My heart is loud, my breathing roughens, I twist my fingers into fists.

'Read this and you can sign it tomorrow.' She gives me an information sheet. 'If you don't sign it we'll have to make you involuntary.'

You will have a general anaesthetic.

A small electric current is passed between two electrodes on your scalp.

When you wake up, you will have no memory of the procedure.

It is completely painless.

While I wait for the first session of ECT I seek out Coby on the couch.

'Have you been to the Philippines?' he asks, his eyes are so blue they might have been scooped out of the sky. 'It's not just the islands. It's the people. And the jungle. Want to listen to some music?' Coby has earphones and a portable CD player. He lends me the left earpiece and we sit together on the couch listening to Chinese opera.

'Chen Shu Liang,' he says, pointing at his cd player.

'You have beautiful eyes Coby,' I say suddenly. He stares at me.

'Laughter always was the best medicine,' he replies, gets up and walks away, earphones trailing behind him. I can't tell if he thinks I'm mocking him.

The ECT room has a trolley bed in the centre, a mobile cupboard full of medication, a defibrillator and a view over the road to the park. I lie down on the bed face up. There's a picture of a forest on the roof. The anaesthetics registrar puts an IV needle in the back of my left hand. The ECT nurse, Anna, lifts up my gown and places ECG markers down the centre of my chest and under my left breast. I feel horribly exposed. Then she puts dobs of Vaseline on my scalp where the electrodes will go; it's cold and sticky. Bernice is talking on her mobile in the corner of the room.

'Ready?' asks Anna.

I nod. Ready to die.

The anaesthetic registrar attaches a syringe to the IV line and begins to push through a white liquid – I can feel it running up the cephalic vein in my arm, heavier than blood, then my head is assaulted with a huge buzzing and the world goes white.

3

'Kate,' a voice is speaking from far above me. I have no idea where I am; I am not even sure who I am. The room is all white – walls, floor, beds, curtains. If this is death, it's whiter than I imagined it.

'You've just had ECT,' says the voice.

'Why am I here?' I ask.

'Kate, you've just had your first ECT.'

I sit up, rip the IV line out of my arm and try to get out of bed over the railings. I struggle with the sheets, I can't feel my feet, I can't remember why I've been arrested, 'What have I done?' I shout. People appear from various directions. 'Don't touch me! Please! No! I haven't done anything wrong.' The world is turning too fast, I am back down on the bed and injected with something that makes everything peculiar and fuzzy.

'You were very confused, we've had to give you some midazolam,' says Anna when I wake up again. I'm still confused. A few hot tears ooze their way out of my red, hot eyes. I am numbed so effectively by the midazolam that I understand why they call it a chemical restraint.

'Do you have a faith?' Anna asks.

'Pardon?'

'Do you believe in God?'

'No.'

'How are you going to heal?' she asks.

'Hammer and nails,' I answer. She takes my hand.

Back on the ward, the music therapist has come in with his guitar for a sing-along. We sit around him in a circle and sing Crowded House, Cat Stevens, Bob Dylan and Gary Jules . . . mad world . . . Linda walks into the room and attempts to sit on his knee.

'Linda, I can't play like this,' he says. 'Sit down over there.'

Linda makes kissing noises, 'Ooh, you're hot!' she says.

The music opens up a kind of conduit between my brain and heart. Even though my back and arms and legs feel like they've been put on the rack and it takes me a whole minute to stand up because of post-ECT muscle spasms, the music – guitar notes and the act of singing – is a flash, then a ray, warm like bath water, almost human.

'Where's your shirt, Coby?' asks Lisa B later, in the main room. He ignores her.

'Coby, you can't walk around without a shirt.' She takes him by the arm and walks him down the corridor to the bedrooms. In the courtyard someone has strung the inside tape of a cassette across the trees from one end of the courtyard to the other. It shimmers and shivers in the breeze like a sudden sculpture. I walk outside slowly and raise my hands in the air in homage.

'Coby and Hana,' says a nurse, walking past fast with a large pair of scissors. It takes them over an hour to get it down; despite their best efforts strings of tape are taken up by the wind, drawn heavenward, are flying; the clouds make a superb backdrop.

Evenings I curl into one of the grey vinyl chairs in front of the TV. Nothing on the television looks familiar. I can't remember ever having seen the newsreaders, I can't understand the news, the stories are foreign and confusing, my eyes won't focus. This is life without punctuation. This is a commentary of rappers whose dance I barely keep up with, round and about they go free as air, they do not acknowledge, but rather breeze through and past and between as though nothing else exists, their hair in my head is quite red, tangled, curling at the ends, mixed with air and light it shimmers. I can't quite grasp them, rein them in, slow them down, they are turning, looking at me, laughing, are gone.

One patient is arguing with another in the hall. 'Just give me a fuckin' cigarette,' the new patient says. 'Just one.'

'Get your own,' the other says.

'Fuckin' bitch.' The new patient walks towards me up the corridor. She's wearing hospital pyjamas several sizes too small, the fat around her hips and abdomen is leaking over the sides, she smells musty, like the aftermath of sex. Her face is large and round and her eyes show sorrow to their very depths and something else – a labyrinthine bewilderment. When she leers at me, she has no teeth.

For the next four weeks, three times a week, the ECT procedure repeats itself: up on the bed, lie down, ECG leads, Vaseline, needle in vein, injection, the cold, the rush, the falling. I hang suspended; I am disembodied; I am nowhere. I am transient as shadow, soon fading and dying, bereft of sun. The kabbalah says 'when a person stands in the light but does not give out light, a shadow is created'.

It's my twenty-sixth birthday. Friends from school, Tanya and Penny, bring red and orange gerberas – small suns in a vase in the sunlight. My parents bring roses and chocolate and books. We sit together in the day room, hunched up on a couch that has long ago lost its stuffing.

'Are you okay?' they ask. My mother looks thinner, my father's hair is greyer and I'm culpable.

'It'll be okay,' I try a creaky smile. An old man with white hair sticking out all over his head and a long white beard sprints the length of the ward stark naked. Three staff are after him, 'Fuck you!' he shouts, disappearing into the courtyard.

Thanks to ECT, memory has left me a soggy trail, mired with half-truths and confusion. Whole days are black holes – the normal neuronal connections that forge new memory stagnate, and with a loss of emotional breadth the entire world encapsulates into the boxy rooms of the ward. I have shed my brain.

In an attempt to make sense of things, I write scratchy notes in the notebooks that I carry everywhere. The notebooks are unlined; writing tracks across the pages like trails of ants in search of food. Some mornings I sit with my dear friend, Tan Ying, in the courtyard and it is all I can do to pronounce her name. I'm astonished that she puts up with me.

The consultant psychiatrist suggests I apply for the Disability Support Pension. 'Best you face facts, Kate,' she says. 'Your sort of illness doesn't go away. It's very unlikely you'll be able to work.'

I stare at her.

'Hey!' Someone shouts outside the consulting room door. 'HDU's on fire!'

I turn slowly just as the sonorous fire alarm sounds. Everyone is milling around the nurses station. The HDU patients are being walked out into the main ward, a nurse at each arm. Most of them are so heavily medicated with phenothiazines that they mince with Parkinsonian steps, arms dead at their sides. We're herded out the front of the psychiatric unit while the fire alarm changes to a more insistent whoop, lingering on the last note. The fire trucks arrive, then the police. There's a vague smell of smoke but no flames. Coby is brought out last between two nurses and two security guards. He looks frail but his eyes are lit with the light of epiphany.

'Florid,' says one of the nurses holding him up. Coby folds onto the ground in his orange flannel pyjamas, his black hair slicked back with brilliantine, his patent leather shoes still on.

Coming back into self after a crisis is as slow as mending bone. Psychiatric illness affects the deep centres of the brain that govern perception, emotion, behaviour and personality. These areas – the prefrontal cortex, the thalamus and limbic system manifest the hidden experience of the mind as opposed to the core motor and sensory functions of the brain.

In the night I slip past the night staff and go out into the courtyard, lie down on a bench and look up at the sky. The night air ripples. According to Scottish mathematician J.S. Haldane, 'the universe is not only queerer than we suppose, but queerer than we can suppose.' This gives me comfort. The stars are out – gleaming cantos of space. In the wide, wide night, there is only the essential smallness of self and the tiny equilibrium of earth and air on which we exist.

Anna finds me occasionally on the ward and we sit side by side on the wooden seats in the courtyard. She has a beautiful face – rich brown eyes that have a depth and an intelligence, liquid soul. She is wise. The people in my head don't know quite what to make of her, they mutter together and flitter, they are edgy.

Another appointment with the plastics people. They take the splint and bandages off. It is odd to see that skin again, the raised dark pink scar like a thick, oily snake, almost circumferential. Disgusting. I go for a walk in the park.

I walk faster.

In the park there are leaves forming on the plane trees, shining with newness. I lie down on the grass, put my face as close to the grass as I can. A small black beetle, brilliant as a mirror is crawling about down there. I watch it travel several centimetres – up over the green stems, falling back down, finding a new way.

Back on the ward Rachel and Simon are playing basketball in the courtyard. The new patient has urinated all over the courtyard bench.

'If she was my dog, I'd shoot her,' says Simon.

She shuffles in her stained pants, asking for cigarettes, picks through the butts on the ground, finds one with a bit of tobacco, asks for a light. No one will give her one.

'You're all mad,' she says. 'Mad.'

Tan Ying brings in my cello and some sheet music. I take the cello out of its case slowly and stroke the brown wood with the back of my hand. It is cool and smooth. I take out the bow with its clean smell of resin. White resin dust gets on my clothes and sticks there like dandruff. I pluck the C string. It resonates even without the bow. I place the cello between my legs and rock back and forth a little and tighten the bow and play an open A and smile. I pick up the sheet music: Bach's first suite for solo violoncello. The music is notes crawling all over the paper, black on white, like ants. I squint, shake my head, turn the page upside down.

'I can't read it,' I say. 'My brain's fried.' Tan Ying offers me comfort; she holds my hand and rubs my back.

The next day I wake up and know immediately I've had enough. There are new cameras in the ceiling – several of them in the air conditioning vents and behind the sprinklers. There may be more. I can't be sure any longer about the motives of staff – if they have been trying to kill me with ECT, with the drugs, the food, for some reason I'm still alive. Do I want to die? If I don't want to die, I have to leave. I stand in the corner of the room – I must be reasonable. The rain runs down the window, gets caught in the throats of the

22

calla lilies. I pack my bag, strip the bed and wait at the nurses' station.

Lisa B listens to my request. I try to speak politely, my hands flutter. 'Can you wait till after the morning meeting?' she asks. 'I need to talk to your doctor.'

'No,' I say, looking up at the cameras. 'I'm ready to go now.'

'Are you voluntary?' she asks.

'Yes.'

'How are you feeling?'

'Oh, good, really good. Much better.' I smile.

'Okay, give me a minute.' Lisa B disappears into the staff area, speaks to the psych reg, walks back out to me. 'You're not on a treatment order, are you?'

'No, no.'

'Have you got enough medication?'

'Plenty of everything,' I say.

'Thanks, Lisa,' I say.

She locks the door behind me.

When I get home there's a message on the answering machine from Anna. I call her, and agree to complete the ECT program as an outpatient, Mondays, Wednesdays, Fridays. I am under no illusion that ECT actually works; I catch the tram to the hospital in the mornings to see Anna and to have a few minutes of oblivion under the anaesthetic. Waking from the anaesthetic I rise up from deep under water and gasp, mouth wide open like a fish, lose all sense of my body, become the floating consciousness. I tell Anna I'm made of bad DNA. She says we all have something that makes us beautiful; we all have a right to be alive. I smile. I don't believe her.

Li, phen, pen, thio, tem, tram. This could be a poem or a piece of music whose notes intone my death. '. . . Send not to know for whom the bell tolls; it tolls for thee.' It tolls for me. I take all of the tablets into the living room and line the bottles and the blister packs up on the floor. My head is clear as water. Bach's fourth cello suite fills the room with sound that is as reassuring as it is magnificent. This is my death. I put on appropriate clothing: jeans, shirt, jumper, socks, no need for shoes. I fill up big bowls of water and food for the cats and give them a kiss on the top of their heads; their fur like silk threads comes away in my mouth.

It is evening. The last lengths of sun are deeply pink on the right of the sky. There is a half moon in the bottom of the sky. I have a jug of water and a glass by the couch and my eyes are full of music and the softness of the sky. Breathing is sweet but finite. The people in my head are quiet, we are all in agreement: it is the right time to die.

I sit on the grey carpet, cross-legged, with my back to the couch. I start with the half bottle of white, coffin-shaped tablets. I take them carefully, two at a time. Then I take the blue ones, the white ones, the yellow ones, the orange ones, the other white ones. It takes about five minutes. I lie on the couch and pull a clean white sheet over me. The phone is off the hook, the lights are out, all the windows are open to let in the fresh air – a room gets very cloying with a dead body in it. I close my eyes and fold my hands neatly over my abdomen.

The room I am in is very dark. The blind covering a window on the left wall lets in a tiny stream of blue light. The bed I am in has high metal sides. There's a woman sitting on a chair in the corner. I try to move and find I can't. I feel my body, finger pads lightly touching, pressing the tube that runs out of my nose, the tube that runs out of my neck, the long electrical cords running from my chest into a monitor that looks like a television. It is very quiet. The woman in the corner is reading a magazine.

The room I am in is very dark. The blind covering a window on the left wall lets in a tiny stream of blue light. The bed I am in has high metal sides. I try to sit up and find I can roll over. Immediately the monitor next to my head starts to bleep and call. The woman on the chair gets up, someone else comes into the room.

'Sorry,' I say. 'Sorry.'

'You're connected to a heart monitor.'

The room I am in is very dark. The blind covering a window on the left wall lets in a tiny stream of blue light. My parents are here and Anna is here and my friend Tanya is here but I can't quite reach them, I am lying underneath a glass wall. How do I move towards them, how do I reach out?

'You are in the Cardiology Unit,' a nurse says one morning. 'Your heart rhythm is irregular. You nearly died, but you're getting better now.'

'I'm alive?'

'Anna and your friend Tanya found you and called an ambulance and came into the hospital with you.' She walks away, out of the room, her shoes squeaking a little on the linoleum.

4

For the following six months I live in a kind of nether world – a dead space. Recovery grinds forwards. Stops. Grinds. My parents arrange for frozen meals to be delivered fortnightly. The fridge is otherwise empty. There are bags of coffee beans and cat food in the cupboard under the sink, and blocks of dark chocolate and dusty, unlabelled spice jars in the pantry, along with packets of pasta and rice and bottles of sauce months past their use-by date.

There is little difference between day and night inside my flat; globes in the living room throw the same light. On the walls Ian Curtis and Nick Drake examine their shoes next to Munch's *Scream* and posters of paintings by Marc Chagall, René Magritte, Picasso, Escher and Albrecht Dürer. They provide sustenance.

Most days I get out of bed in the late morning, shuffle to the kitchen for coffee, sit on the floor in the living room with the cats and coffee and medical textbooks, poetry, British crime fiction, books by de Beauvoir, Nietzsche, Camus, Jung. Books to keep me alive. Books that remain closed and still on the floor.

The phone rings, the air shifts, I blink.

In the afternoon I eat a block of kosher chocolate with hazelnuts. There are words on the wrapper in French and Hebrew and English, equally unintelligible. I screw the wrapper up and the cats shiver it around the room with the tips of their paws.

The phone rings, the air shifts, I blink.

Once the sun goes down it's safe to leave the flat and I walk in the dark down the street to buy chocolate and merlot and a newspaper for the pictures and headlines. It takes over an hour to look at the pictures and read the headlines.

Then there's the cocktail of evening medication that induces sedation but not necessarily sleep. If one thinks of sleep as having a role in cognitive and emotional processing, then dreaming is a reflection of the mind's attempt to evaluate and reorganise emotion and memory. If dreams are a portal to the inner world of the psyche, then I am preoccupied with Sacrifice, Death, Primal Thinking and the essential Red of Blood. To keep the people in my head from taking over, I play music from the good stereo in the living room through the night. Every morning I'm surprised to be alive.

The people who live in my head are elusive. There are many secrets. They inhabit the body, the brain – but are not me. They have a consciousness (of sorts) but are without corporeal form. It doesn't seem to bother them. There are days when I soak up colour and sound in different dimensions and life is serene, other times there is silence, or howling – not a scream – deeper and drawn out, more guttural.

Henry is the closest thing to humane. He has a richness, a gentility. He is thoughtful and moderate. Henry is married to Rose. Rose, woman of valour. Rose is enveloping warmth, flowers, perfume, flowing clothes – chiffon and velvet – all colour.

The Cold Ones are severe. Unrelenting. Psychopathic in their gleeful execution of pain. They are clever. They sneer, undermine, are disdainful. They prefer to whisper – criticisms and threats. They are featureless, blank-faced. They do not blink or flinch. They like shadow.

The Savage Ones are fire and brute force. They roar in the imperative.

you bitch do this this

The Cold Ones nod.

shes scared now

They titter and slither and whisper in the shadows.

KILL HER

The Savage Ones like rape. They're not averse to fights, assault, blood, death. They find it funny. They make me dream it. They like to hear things crack and wrench. Red eyes. Red skin. Heat. Sweat.

Then there are the Cruel Ones – fond of knives and teeth.

touch us you die

They're always moving, they don't sleep. The Cruel Ones and the Savage Ones gang up. Hilarious to bind hands and eyes, to dart about, to whisper, to kick where there is tenderness, to snicker where there is pain. To shout obscenities, entice nightmares, scream (shrilly); lose all sense of light and dark.

you are rotting bitch rotting we are gutting you like a fish

They are gleeful.

don't move don't breathe don't fucking breathe suffocate there is force in circumstance BITCH stab yourself you're a fucking animal we're watching you bleed where's the red we're gonna kill you (singsong, lilting) do you deserve this

Yes.

Sometimes my parents come around and open mail and pay bills and help me clean. Without them I'd be heading for destitute. We go to a local cafe for lunch. Everything outside in the day is moving 40 per cent too fast for my eyes to process. I keep my head down. The first item on the menu is French onion soup. Three words, French and Onion and Soup. Come on, I say to myself. Nothing. The words have drowned somewhere between my occipital lobe (vision) and parietal lobe (visuospatial processing). I look up. In the cafe people are chatting, laughing, eating. I look at the menu. Nothing. Don't you dare cry. I pinch the loose skin on my abdomen. The waiter arrives.

'Hi,' he says. 'How are you today?'

'Very well thanks,' I say, smiling. 'How are you?'

He smiles back. 'What can I get for you?'

'French onion soup, please,' I say pleasantly. I may as well have ordered tripe.

Recovery grinds forwards. Stops. Grinds. One step forward, two steps back, then one forward and one back, then two forward and one back. Many people recover partially after an episode of acute illness and are then stuck with a background level of disability that is life-long. For some, the background disability gets worse with every acute episode.

Friends from university, Tan Ying and Lara and Melyse, are completing their hospital internships, moving into responsible working lives and climbing Abraham Maslow's hierarchy of needs. They are experimenting with love. Their clothes are crisp and their bodies shine. I am now able to pick up the phone at home and answer it when it rings.

Overnight my hair has grown and greyed. The season has changed. With some return of cognitive function, the other side of life materialises: the external realm, a kind of ocean on the surface of which I flap about like an insect. Periodically I swim. Periodically I drown. The swimming requires negotiation. Every day I'm new to the water and the water does not part to welcome me. It is deep and dark and cold.

I revise for hours from clinical textbooks, terrified that I've lost years of knowledge secondary to ECT. I go out with friends, nod and laugh in the right places. I care very much about the happenings in their lives and my stupid fucking heart is cold.

Then one morning the sun reaches through the top of the curtains, setting the bedroom ceiling singing like water. I breathe and smile – a true smile – the first for almost a year. Something warm is inside me and I get up and the warmth is energy and it's in my legs and belly and it's part of that weird, nebulous thing called pleasure.

The people in my head hiss and jeer–

die die

But today, I think I might get through this. I just might.

5

The blue of the sky is what I think about most. The blue of the sky, and the pale spring sun and the budding trees. It is a time for renewal, for stretching out old bones, stepping into the light. I examine the unfolding of spring in my little garden. The infinite awe of the universe has exploded into a purple and white magnolia; there is a blush on the ground at my feet. In the house the walls suck in sunlight and lift themselves up into the ceiling. Clothing dries in the breeze, mould lifts off old shoes, mould spores dissolve in the sun, disperse in air fragrant with plum blossom.

The people in my head are slightly feverish whenever the season changes. Henry and Rose magnify space, Rose is forever smoothing her dresses, taking steps to the left, to the right, hearing her fabric swish and curl. Henry is compassionate about her need to show off. He follows a pace or two behind, he takes her hand, kisses it, touches her hair with the tips of his fingers. Rose has a ring on her index finger – a garnet set in rose-gold filigree. She knows how to make it catch the light, to make the garnet a ruby. She can sit and let the light reflect off a facet of garnet onto the wall, let it dance there.

Molten metal couldn't be more beautiful than this, says Rose from her rocking chair, the toes of one bare foot resting on the floor. Henry is sitting in between her legs. She is brushing his long hair that is black and straight as water.

Slower, he says. She slows. She makes the hair breathe, it comes alive, like light through a dark lampshade, it glows. *Beautiful,* says Rose, and sighs.

The other people in my head sneer—

pathetic

They sound like wind through long grass.

paaath kill her

They want Rose dead as much as they want me dead, and yet we aren't good company. Rose and Henry know how to make me cringe, they know where there is softness, where my heart lives.

6

A research assistant position in clinical cancer research is advertised in the paper. 'Clinical' means working with patients, for which I have trained for six years. As an assistant I would not have primary responsibility for someone's medical care. This I consider essential because of the risk that I might become unwell again and with it lose the ability to think rationally. So I apply for the job and commence full-time work six months after discharge from hospital.

The new work environment is a small team of clinical researchers located in a busy public hospital. They're trialling a variety of new treatments for cancer – new kinds of chemotherapy, radiotherapy, immunotherapy and the very first gene-targeted biological agents. My role will be in patient education and support and in the collection of data that will later be used in statistical analysis.

Participation by patients in a clinical trial is entirely voluntary. I learn how best to talk with people about complex medical science so that it becomes accessible and understandable. I learn to observe body language, to ask open questions and to be comfortable with silence.

The other members of the team are warm and welcoming and the work is challenging without being stressful. I WILL NOT fuck up this opportunity to be part of the normal working world, to contribute something.

Appearing 'normal' is an hour-by-hour challenge. To get to work on time I set the alarm for five. It takes over an hour to wake up because of the sedating effects of alcohol and evening medication. Out of bed, espresso, shower, black and grey clothes two sizes too big, more medication, espresso, train, office. I take an interest in my colleagues' lives, work hard, avoid conflict, follow instructions.

The people in my head are quieter; they hiss and slither. If they start to get loud, I curl my hands into fists to keep the rest of my body language in check and then I engage with something or someone else – anything as a distraction, anything so I don't have to listen to their bile. If the creeping feeling of paranoia makes it hard to breathe, I walk for a while in the local park – off the paths, under the fig trees.

In the evening there's European chocolate for dinner and then I unfurl into bed amongst layers of pyjamas and quilts and blankets and cats. I don't cry. Sometimes I howl.

Tonight Melyse and her boyfriend James and I are pre-gig-drinking. Nick Cave and the Bad Seeds are playing at Festival Hall, a venue known as Melbourne's grungy House of Stoush because it was originally built for boxing and wrestling matches. Music keeps those parts of me that are commonly called heart and soul alive – alive in the way a leafless shrub has still-green inside some of its brown twigs. (As a child this discovery gave me a rush of joy. 'It's not dead yet!' I'd shout. 'I'll save you I'll save you,' to the plant in its pot by the door, nearly dead. The smallness of the world). Music does this religious-like thing of thrusting me skyward. Going to a concert is the closest I'll ever come to flying.

Me and Melyse are in the statutory uniform for the evening: black skirts, black t-shirts, black boots, black hair, black fingernails. She looks fabulous. Inside the hall we're drinking Coopers Pale Ale, watching all the other people in black – older, younger, thin, not-so, smoking, drinking. Smoke from the smoke machine makes me wheeze.

The lights go out and it's so dark, no breathing and then 'Yeeeaaaah,' everyone shouts, and they're here, six men on stage: guitar, bass, drums, percussion, keyboard and Nick in his black suit, spider-walking and smoking. Black. The bass. And that voice. Fuck. Sandpaper, honey, a deep tolling bell, guts everywhere. Piano now and someone playing a violin like a guitar and I'm on the ceiling hotcoldhot arms sweat my head is burning the shivering delicious this measuring of truth the violin the violin harder, reaching in with that red beat, hot like eyes are, you and me Nick, finally. Hah. Fantasy is a fine thing.

Whisky is my new evening friend. From the moment I come home from work it is waiting for me, waiting in its glass bottle, pure amber, pure abandon, oblivion. The first drink, a thick slop of whisky and ice is all flurry, all the taste, the fine smoothness, the fire as it goes down the gullet. The second is softer, there's a haze in the room, the walls are further away, there is less leering. Inside my head the scuffling ceases. The third is softer still and warm and calm is seeping in. My eyes blur. *Mercy*, whispers Henry.

death

But they whisper. The fourth drink and I am aware of the spirit, holy or otherwise, residing outside my window. It is the darkness of a soul, the brightness of a camellia, the softness of pussy willow. It sits in the silver birch playing a tune in a minor key. With its wings folded it breathes whitely on the glass. I stretch out towards it, whisky bottle at my side. The fifth drink and I leave the room, crawl up the stairs with my eyes closed, I lie on the stairs, arms above my head, face drizzled with whisky and spittle, jumper around my neck. I keen.

Weekends I am dried up, thick and fuzzy, voice muffled, foul smelling. I put on my clothes carefully, socks last, mindful to bend over slowly to avoid vomiting. I pick up the whisky bottle and drink what's left, holding it up for the last drops. *Mercy*, whispers Henry. *Death*, whisper the others.

The local bottle shop isn't open till 10 a.m. I find some beer in the cupboard and drink that. There are magpies calling outside. I sit on the couch drinking beer and listen to the magpies. I take a lot of Largactil and some clonazepam left over from the hospital and curl up tight tight on the floor. I stay that way for a long time. The magpies stop calling.

7

Each week I have an appointment at the local Community Mental Health Clinic. It is a hot spring. The asphalt radiates heat, black and thick. Birds and people move slower. Leaves, wilted, move slower in the slow breeze. There are no clouds. The Community Clinic is housed in a building owned by the electricity company; it is an incongruous spot at the front, a blemish. Mad people come here.

Michael greets me in the same way every week: 'Hi Kate, will you marry me?'

'Hi Michael,' I say. 'No.'

'Why not?'

'I don't want to marry anyone right now.'

'Okay. Who are you here to see? Me?'

'Helen.' Michael goes outside to have another cigarette, shoulders slumped, perfectly baldhead round as a sun in the sunlight. Later he pulls up a chair and sits facing me in the waiting room, legs spread, his knees reaching the sides of my chair.

'Michael,' says someone from behind the desk, 'that's inappropriate.' He sighs heavily and pushes his chair back. He has the darkest brown eyes and he hardly ever blinks.

Helen calls me from the door to the offices. We walk together down the long corridor, tiny rooms to either side just big enough for two chairs and perhaps a desk. Helen is a psychologist and case-manager. Her role is to provide a single point of contact for the outpatient clients (and carers) of a public mental health service.

'How are you?' Helen asks, sitting down and arranging her floral skirt around her knees. I look up at the ceiling for cameras. The people in my head pour into my left ear—

kill her we said kill her do it do it

I hold my hands tight together so the knuckles go white and the fingers blue.

'Okay. Yes, okay,' I say. I hunch my shoulders a little. Helen is adept at using silence as a means of communication. She waits.

'Well, at least I'm not in hospital,' I say.

'Yes. What have you been doing?'

'Drinking.' I look at the floor; find a stain pattern on the carpet that looks like a flower.

'How much are you drinking?'

'Half a bottle of Scotch . . . over an evening and a night.'

'Why?'

'Keeps my head in check. All the spewing . . . shit.'

'What would happen if you didn't drink?'

'I'd go mad.'

John died today. Sensitive, funny John. Married, two kids John. Musician John. Small-business owner John. We met at a personal development course several years ago (an almost-cult) with lots of hitting and banging things and shouting, but we survived that, and Shaz and Zoë and I and John and Andrew and others formed enduring friendships. Our beautiful St Kilda friend hanged himself today.

Dear John, all the things we want to say, all the things you need to hear . . . here we are tonight, sitting in a tight, urgent circle, one by one trying to explain what you mean to us; which parts of your soul we managed to glimpse; why we've all failed you so badly. The sun throws its red-gold light across the water, and I ache that you do not feel the warmth on your arms and face. I'll be looking for you along Fitzroy Street – your guitar, a bright orange shirt and your smile.

Back home in the very early morning and I can't sleep, so I sit in bed with the cats and the tears that fall and fall and write for him.

The weekends pass, blurred into half-consciousness, unconsciousness and small periods of extraordinary white light when I manage to walk to the bottle shop. Whether as a result of ECT or as a result of acute illness or some combination of the two, I can't recall addresses of friends, passwords, bank account details. And I can't remember where I might have written them down before I went into hospital. It is odd to be able to remember the serial white cell counts of a patient, to be able to explain to a colleague the histological subtypes of melanoma, and yet not to know whether my parents' phone number begins with a 5 or an 8. It is odd, but it is explainable: I have a kind of retrograde amnesia, common after ECT. It means I can lay down new memory fine, but I've lost some old memory and I have to relearn the simplest things.

So this outer shell of Kate, a foreign entity, is a careful observer, a careful mimic, paralleling appropriate behaviour in the presence of others. It runs a tight ship during the workday and it negotiates social events like a rather comely old lady. With every ocean wave falling on it, the outer shell presses out another layer, re-moulds itself, sets.

Most of the rest of me is crossing the divide from existentialism to nihilism. Nietzsche knew all about nihilism: our existence (action, suffering, willing, feeling) has no meaning. Existence without intrinsic value. Black cloth, the cloth of death, of funerals, the

a Villanelle
for John.

~~The river~~ ~~Dear John~~ –
<u>Where we took our vows</u>

I passed the place ^where^ ~~we~~ we took our vows.
The bluestone walls ~~as~~ were falling ~~down~~.
The moon still shines, the water flows.

We ~~tried~~ tried to understand his vows,
the experts mistook his many griefs.
I ~~passed~~ the place where we ~~took~~ our vows.

They shocked his unwieldy neurones back.
Then tied him down to make him stay.
The moon still shines, the water flows.

His family disappeared, as time allows,
We were ~~left~~ with ~~the~~ pills, the moon +
                                          stars
I passed the place where we ~~took our~~
                                       vows.

there were times the blackness left all
                        but his toes
which remained inexplicably, ~~old~~ frigid
                        + cracked.
The moon still shines, the water flows.

When we found him there, stript of his foes
we lay beside him through the night.
~~the silence and ??~~
I passed the place where we took our vows,
the moon still shines, the water flows
            Vale John, ~~????????~~. Vale.

cloth of death. Time stretches inside the shell as a desert does – distant, uncharted, wide and flat as ice. There is no calm.

'John died,' I tell Helen. 'He was . . . vibrant. I mean really. He kind of shined. He had two gorgeous children. See what depression does? It wrecks families. And the tree out the front of the clinic, the crepe myrtle, has new flowers, did you see it?'

'I'm very sorry,' Helen says.

'The incongruity.'

'Yes.'

'And the injustice. I don't get it.'

We sit. The air doesn't move either.

'Grief is so visceral, you know? There's that moment when you first wake up and it hits you like a fist, right in the centre of the chest.'

'Yes.'

We sit. Both of us here and not here.

'How are you managing at work?' asks Helen after a while.

'Oh. If the worlds stay nice and separate.'

'Tell me about that.'

'The researcher-doctor-person is focused and measured and normal and knowledgeable. We all have some kind of professional front, right? I guess mine is this whole other individual squashed into the bony skeleton, inside the shell but beside, not of, myself.'

'Mmm,' says Helen. 'Is that tiring?'

'Most days I end up on the floor of a toilet cubicle.'

'So it must be a relief to come home at the end of the day?'

'Doesn't matter, the darkness is always there.'

Helen sits quite still, she sits with the darkness, she doesn't try to brush it aside. The darkness oozes into the room.

'Are you sleeping?' she asks.

'Some,' I say. 'Till the dreams . . .'

'Dreams?'

I tell her about the dreams. Most nights the dreams have a theme: barbed wire is hacked across my face, the blood that runs from my forehead is so red and thick and warm that it blocks up my nose and mouth and causes me to choke. I am hit from behind so that I fall forward onto the concrete floor and am left there and it is so cold that my teeth clench into each other and my elbows are numb. The room I am in has no light. I know there will be a knife and I try to curl into a ball, my arms are bound behind me with wire that is prodding the veins on the back of my hands, my head is wrenched back, I am choking, I am probably naked, there is dirt in my eyes, I can't tell if I'm crying, I feel white and helpless as a newborn, there's the iron taste of blood, and salt and grit, the acute sound of a hammer on metal, the sudden cold of metal on the skin of my back and the only accompaniment is laughter – gleeful, mirthless.

'Are you thinking about harming yourself?' Helen asks.

'Most days.' (Every day). I smile.

'I'll arrange for review with a psychiatrist.' She takes my hand and puts it between both of hers. She has small hands; her palms are soft and dry and warm.

I walk out into the Community Clinic waiting area. People are playing pool in the corner of the room. There are posters up on the walls about schizophrenia, panic disorder, depression and mania. There are empty polystyrene coffee cups on the floor and bits of newspaper. Someone has been painting with watercolours and has left paints in a mess of yellow and blue on the table. A young woman sits waiting, the skin of her hands pink as a sunset. She has almost no hair except for some fine, long wisps near the base of her skull and on the very top of her head. She is reading a book of poetry – I can tell it's Emily Dickinson by the use of long dashes.

Outside the heat of the day lifts up from the ground. There is a strong northerly wind, the branches of the trees bear down and the leaves rattle. I walk home. The people in my head have begun to comment on my movements.

now she's brushing her hair now she's getting dressed wasted breath ugly fucking ugly

I don't look in mirrors. I'm terrified of the sight of my body, of its pathetic mass of flesh, scars like red infestations under the skin of my arms and legs. I haven't looked at my body for several years, I shower with my eyes closed, towel dry with my eyes closed.

Hippocrates described melancholia (black bile) as a state of 'despondency, sleeplessness, irritability, and restlessness.' A depressive episode can last longer than a year without effective treatment. Even with treatment, many people like me continue to experience 'sub-syndromal' symptoms in between episodes of acute illness. These are by definition less severe, but they complicate day-to-day life.

To those lucky enough not to have experienced it, depression may appear selfish. Depression is not selfish. It's a barren well, deep and dark, and you're alone right at the bottom of it and there is no light at the top of the well so you cannot see beyond your own suffering. After weeks, months, sometimes years in the well you lose even the basest urges of life: hunger, thirst, sleep, libido, hygiene, health, social contact, order.

Theories for the causes of depression include aggression turned inward, object loss, learned helplessness, negative cognitive schemata and neurochemical imbalance. It is probably a combination of these as well as genetics; all under the influence of personality.

you are rotting

I am rotting; my innards are turning brown-grey like the

decomposition of the dead. Soon there will be nothing left inside me except air and water.

I meet with Jim, the psychiatrist, Friday evening after work. He is balding, has a slight paunch and a youthful face. He wears a suit; his shoes are polished. He asks me the usual battery of questions: appetite, sleep, sadness, pleasure, energy, somatic symptoms, psychotic symptoms, suicide. He leans back in his chair with his legs crossed and his arms folded over his chest.

'What medication are you on?' He asks.

'Venlafaxine and lithium.'

'Let's add mirtazapine 30 mg and some clonazepam at night,' he says. 'See you next week.' I walk away with the prescriptions and a hole in my heart.

Simon is sitting in the waiting room, hunched in a large brown coat, big boots on his feet. He looks hunted. 'Simon?' I say. His eyes are deeply black all the way through, there's hardly any white. He doesn't recognise me, or perhaps can't. I need a bath. I smell like sweat and whisky and cigarettes. Back home I take some sandal-wood incense (such an aromatic smoke) and I take the flame (the blue and yellow light) and I atone atone. Flame on pale skin goes red then white then black, always in the same order. Will the perfume linger?

Morning. Light drifts in with the dust motes. It is already warm. The lion-cat is stretched out at the end of the bed, his convex belly moving up and down rhythmically with his breath. My fingers are sore and swollen, skin reddened with white and black holes where the incense burned in.

kill yourself shriek coffin worth the price die bitch shrieeek we're killing you

I keep my head low to avoid the internal blows and walk out into the sunlight with hot coffee, holding the cup between thumb and index finger. There are honeyeaters in the potato plant and a wattlebird in the red flowers of the grevillea. I stand quite still, watching them.

By 11 p.m. Sunday evening it is no longer possible to ignore the normal tasks required for the looming normal week. Wash clothes. Grocery shopping – chocolate, cat food, cat milk and a pair of supermarket flannel pyjamas. Wash self. Wash hair. Dry self. Dry hair. Dry clothes. Breathe. Set alarms.

'Have you ever fallen in love, Kate?' Helen asks the following week.

'With other minds, oh yes. Many times. Right now for example . . . with ee cummings and Matsuo Bashō. And I've fallen in love with other souls – twice.'

'What about with all of another person, someone you actually know?'

'I don't think so. Not physically. Not with another body.'

'Did you ever have a high school crush?'

'Yep,' I smile, remembering.

'With whom?'

I flush. 'Virginia Woolf.'

Helen smiles. Then she says, 'Do you think that's unusual?'

'I don't know. Is it? Reading her journals and her fiction kept me alive.'

'Yes, but *she* isn't alive.'

Later I wander down the corridor for another review with Jim. Another battery of questions, to which I give the same answers.

Yes, I have trouble sleeping.

Yes, I'm drinking too much.

Yes, I have trouble concentrating.

No, I don't have visions.

No, I don't hear voices that other people can't hear.

Yes, I think a lot about dying.

No, I can't cry.

He doesn't notice the burns on my hands; he keeps his arms and legs folded into himself as before. 'We'll increase the mirtazapine,' he says. 'Double it.' He smoothes his hair and ushers me out of the room. I leave with another prescription and walk to the bottle shop for more whisky.

shoot yourself bitch shoot yourself you're dying anyway

I walk faster. Wild Turkey, Jack Daniels, Canadian Club, Jim Beam, Famous Grouse, Woodstock, Ballentine's. It rains. Hard clear drops of water hit the warm ground and sizzle; the smell of hot asphalt rises into the air. I buy 700 ml of Wild Turkey and walk home in the rain. By the fifth drink I'm floating on the roof, up there with the daddy-long-legs and wisps of web, up there with Rose and Henry and the unholy spirit.

My little finger starts flickering first. Little tiny muscle fasciculations flick flick pause flick flick. Then my ring finger flick flick pause. Like they are keeping time. Like I have suddenly developed a sort of Parkinson's disease. I hear them at night rustling the sheets; I feel them carrying on their own little dance. Flickering.

Hana sits with Simon in the Community Clinic smoking area, curled up in yellow tights and a floral dress, her black hair catching the light, grey eyes pooling the light. When she speaks her voice is a low cadence.

'The consumer liaison group,' she says. 'I'm thinking of joining.'

'Yeah?' says Simon.

'Yeah, because of the wards, and here. I haven't seen the same guy here more than twice. I'm sick of having to repeat my history every bloody consultation.'

'I got assaulted on the ward last time I was in,' says Simon. 'Some guy in HDU tried to strangle me. Big bastard too.'

'What happened?' I ask.

'The music therapist was playing Bob Dylan, then this guy comes up behind me and puts his hands around my neck and squeezes. The music therapist and another patient hauled him off me, not before I'd turned blue. They called a Code Grey and stuck him in seclusion; he was out again the next day. Sick bastard.'

'We've gotta do something about patient safety,' says Hana. 'From the ground up, you know, like a union.'

I walk down the rabbit warren of brown corridors. Jim asks the same questions and increases the dose of mirtazapine by another 30 mg. On the way home my right hand starts to twitch. I lie in bed at night and listen to my foot and my hand and my fingers. Later my leg begins jerking from the knee down and pools of muscle contract in my back like ripples on a body of water.

garrotte garrotte garrotte the world will spin you into obsidian oblivion keep the fires burning watch yourself muddy red

'There's something wrong with my glasses,' I say to the optometrist. 'I can't read the newspaper. At all.'

'Since when?'

'Yesterday.'

'Suddenly?'

'I think it's getting worse.'

He looks closely at the glasses, holds them sideways, holds them up to the light.

'I can't see a problem,' he says. 'I'll examine your eyes if you'd like, but I think you'd be better off seeing a doctor.'

'I am a doctor,' I say, irritably.

'And you're shaking,' he says.

'Sorry. It's these bloody glasses.'

The city is still warm in the very late evening. The sky has merged between grey and brown, heavy with cloud. There are ducks in the water of the river and ducks sitting on the grass along the riverbank. I walk to gain some perspective. I'm sweating. I can take only the smallest mincing steps. A couple of children come down to the river bank with their parents to feed the ducks pieces of bread; with their bright clothing and shining hair they make a counterpoint to the brown of the river. Most of the ducks take off in fright.

Across from the river people gather outside the arts centre after a concert, milling in small groups in filmy evening clothes, I catch the laughter and wonder about it. Over the bridge there is a small ferris wheel moving slowly on its arc, lighting the plane trees yellow and pink against the night sky.

In the morning I visit my GP, Jenny. I sit in the waiting room sweating with both legs jerking unrhythmically. I feel like a marionette.

'Your blood pressure's awfully high. Your pulse is 140,' says Jenny.

I look at the roof and then at her fuzzy figure and there's sweat running down my face like tears.

'What are we going to do about these jerks – this myoclonus?' she asks.

I try to shrug my shoulders.

'Is it getting worse?'

I half-cough-half-retch. My head stutters. 'I'm not . . . I'm sorry, I'm not managing,' I say.

Jenny takes one of my nasty, smelly hands in both of hers. 'Hospital,' she says. 'I'm going to call an ambulance.'

'Oh shit. Shit.'

watch bitch you killer KILLER

The ambulance gurney slides through the Emergency Department doors and I'm assailed by fluorescent light. The ambos deposit me on a trolley in a cubicle where I wait, lying on my back. I lie quietly, thinking. Sometimes I am of the sea – the undercurrent unwinds me. My arms gather together and unfurl, gather and unfurl, held or lulled apart by notes played over and deep under the green-blue water. I have no soul to call my own. That which was, dives with the waves, is tossed amongst seaweed and breathes, breathes, briny water. My bones are brittle as shells. Molluscs covet my ears. A cerise squid engorges my mouth so its tentacles blow like jelly through my lips.

'Kate?' A man in a white coat stands at the end of my bed; four others stand around him, in shorter white coats.

'What's been happening?' he asks. I tell him about the twitches and jerks starting in my little finger and now involving my arms and legs and back and neck, and the sweating and the tremor and the terribly blurred vision. 'I can't walk in a straight line.' My voice is gargled. He moves up to the head of the bed and flicks me suddenly in the centre of the forehead with his thumb and index finger. An onslaught of muscle contractions follows, am I having a grand mal seizure? He leaves the cubicle, taking his students with him, pulling the curtain behind him.

'What do you think of that?' I can hear him talking clearly.

'Epilepsy?' says someone.

'MS?'

'Hypermitotic brain lesion?'

'Metabolic disorder?'

'Meningitis?'

'OD?'

'She said she hadn't OD'd.'

'She could be lying.' They walk away.

Breathing: the low moan of breath, the treacle-thick air, resistant lungs crack at the impact. And the heartbeat: muddy-red, red like ochre after rain, slow, fickle. It goes on despite the mind, to spite the mind. Spiteful. And the mind: thick with the grief of the god-awful awareness of existence. And pain: reaching out from the heart, down from the breast to the belly, to the pelvis, the deepest innards. Nestling there, nesting.

The jerking slows down, finally stops. I lie still. A nurse comes in, takes my blood pressure and temperature, inserts a needle in a vein in my hand, connects it to bag of normal saline and pins it up on a pole over my head. I say thanks; she smiles. The hospital is full of its usual noises: the ping of IV pumps, pagers, the squeak of trolleys on linoleum, people calling one another, the swish of cubicle curtains. A Code Grey is called to the psychiatry wing: threat of assault without a weapon. Someone is paranoid or panicked or in terror.

8

The experience of psychosis is an individual one. Oliver Sacks calls it a state where 'the world is taken apart, undermined, reduced to anarchy and chaos'. R.D. Laing calls it 'the only rational way of coming to terms with an insane world'. I call it a misapprehension of the nature of reality; a blurring of the line between what is Self and what is Other. At its basest level psychosis is terror because sound erupts through the ears into the mind, touch painfully ripples the hairs on skin, breath and voice drive the fantastical figures that float in the night in strange and unbalanced packs, and all nourish paranoia.

Later in the day I am admitted to the neuropsychiatric unit. Rose and Henry have disappeared – I am left with the others, full of bile and phlegm. They scream. I am creating shadow while there is light, and then in darkness, I am nothing. To be locked outside the heart of things – the air, the trees, the sky – is this life? Is nothingness a purity of the soul?

Neuropsychiatry sits at the clinical interface of psychiatry and medicine, focusing on brain-behaviour relationships. Do I have an organic illness or a functional one? Do I have a brain tumour? Am I mad? An electrode is clipped onto my forearm for an electromyogram (EMG) – a recording of the nerve signals in muscles. I'm told to relax or contract my arm; I'm flicked again and again on the forehead, setting off cascades of jerking and twitching. Jim from the clinic visits, sits at the end of my bed for five minutes. He decides to cease the venlafaxine in case I have Serotonin Syndrome.

Outside my window I can see a school and a church and a park where people are carrying on with the beauty of ordinary life. I lie in bed at night and watch the flowers on the curtains of my room wander up and down on the fabric in the half-light afforded by the lit corridor. I can't tell if their wandering signals a problem with my brain or my eyes.

The central nervous system is a finely tuned maze of nerve fibres and neurotransmitters. It controls not only motor and sensory function, breathing and blood pressure, but is also the seat of our personality, our desires, and our capacity to love and to harness creative energy. The nervous system is integral to daily survival, as well as to our ability to communicate and to how we understand the world and ourselves.

Fiona is my roommate in the neuropsych ward. She has Huntington's chorea – a genetic degenerative disease affecting a part of the brain called the basal ganglia. Fiona sits on her bed in the morning and applies lipstick in a loud wiggly line around her mouth. Photos of her children are propped up on her bedside table. She hasn't seen them for two months – not since she took an overdose of paracetamol and codeine while they were in her care. Her husband won't bring them in to see her. He doesn't visit either. Huntington's chorea has an inexorable course through chorea (jerking, writhing) to pneumonia, heart failure, dementia and death. When Fiona is discharged, she'll be transferred to a nursing home. She's 34 years old.

'I'm forgetting everything,' she says as we sit together on the lurid green couch in the day room. 'I'm a walking sieve!' We laugh. She has put her red cardigan on inside out, her ankles stick out from underneath her pyjamas, pale and vulnerable, her speech is slurred and every so often one arm or a leg contorts to the side, a sudden violent movement.

Medical staff send me off to have an electroencephalogram (EEG). First vaseline is dabbed over my scalp reminding me uncomfortably of ECT, then a thousand tiny electrodes are clamped on my skin; I must look like a modern medusa. Alpha waves are recorded when I close my eyes and beta waves when I'm asked to count backwards by 7 from 100, which I struggle with, the people in my head offering their black bile, and my muscles twitching at random.

The ward has people with epilepsy, young people who have had strokes, older people with Parkinson's disease and others, like myself, on whom a diagnosis hasn't been made. We exist in a bubble of illness as though the meaning of our whole lives is to be found within this one space and this one time.

Meaning.

Illness.

The beauty of ordinary life.

9

It is several days before I realise, suddenly and horribly, that I'm missing work. I ring my manager. She says my father called last week. Oh, thank you. Thank you. The relief, like sinking into warm water. Dr David S, grey hair, sombre blue eyes, walks into our room and sits in the chair at the foot of my bed. His nose is slightly bent; he touches it with just the tips of his fingers.

'What are you angry about?' he asks. I look at him in surprise. He doesn't elaborate. I sit very still after he has gone, the people in my head crowding out mature thought. The jerks and twitches have dissipated somewhat so that I feel more like a human being. The following day I'm discharged. A diagnosis for the myoclonus is never made, or at least, never communicated to me.

Outside the hospital everything is moving fast: the wind, the cars, the trams, the people. I'm disorientated; I've been let into the light after a period in the darkness and my legs still won't work. They take malignant little steps, a half-shuffle, a sort of sashay sideways except that I'm not trying to dance. The intimate neuronal coupling between brain and legs that is required for walking – the sensorimotor cortex, the brainstem, spinal cord, the spinal nerves and peripheral nerves and motor neurons and skeletal muscle – appears to have been somewhat abused.

I mince awfully slowly through the park where dogs are running into the wind and kids are playing soccer. The grass under my feet is short and springy though there are patches of dirt where no grass has grown since the winter football season. I sit down under a plane tree. The Buddha of Compassion, Avalokiteshvara, has eleven heads and a thousand arms. On the palms of his thousand hands is an eye, each of which radiates the gaze of compassion across the primordial universe. I often think of him sitting beneath a tree with his thousand arms, as the Buddha himself sat beneath the Bodhi tree, the sacred fig with its heart-shaped leaves.

The plane tree has an exfoliating grey trunk and knobbly joints; its leaves are maple-like, with lobes ending in spiky tips that are greener than the grass at my feet. Sunlight filters through the leaves, throwing their veins into silhouette.

kill yourself kill

I think about this. I think about my death, about where I might die, how I might die and about my body at the time of death– the stench, the bacteria, the excrement. I know what the brain looks like after death; I know what the heart looks like after death. I've stood in the mortuary of the hospital and assisted with the slow dissection of a human being, the removal of the lungs, the liver and spleen, the fragile brain – the seat of humanity. I've smelt the smell of death and seen death on the faces of those who have died, the body finally released. For a long time I sit under the tree. Shadows lengthen. Dogs bark. The street fills with cars. The wind picks up and ruffles the grass. The air is full of the smells of the city. I breathe. I am still. I think of Avalokiteshvara until it gets cold and darkness gathers. Then I shuffle home, Rose and Henry by my side.

To explain the six-day stay in hospital and the funny walking, I tell my manager and workmates that I've had an unusual reaction to one of my asthma meds. It's another four weeks before co-ordination returns. Thankfully, it's easier to get away with funny walking in a hospital, even as a staff member. I avoid other public places including the supermarket. This disconnection between brain and musculature is a most unwelcome reminder of my most unwelcome body.

Michael is sitting in a green vinyl chair in front of the Community Clinic in the late afternoon, smoking.

'Hello Kate,' he says. 'Will you marry me?'

'Hi Michael,' I say. 'No, I won't marry you.'

'Oh. Are you here to see me?'

'Helen and Jim.'

'Can I walk in with you?'

'Sure.' He stubs out his cigarette and loops my arm in his and we shuffle up the stairs together.

'Can I sit with you?' he asks.

'Sure,' I say. He pulls two chairs up close; we sit down, knees touching. He takes off his cap, leans forward, 'I'm pretty smart. I live with my mum but she's good, she's good, yeah, she's good. She is. Want to shoot some pool?' He gets up, puts his cap back on and walks over to the pool table, whose green felt has almost all frayed away. I go to join him but Helen calls me from the entrance to the offices and I follow her down the passageway.

'What do you think caused the shakes?' Helen asks.

'Iatrogenic,' I say.

She raises her eyebrows.

'Too much medication,' I say.

'Where do we go from here?'

'Round in a circle.'

She leans back in her chair, folds her fingers together under her chin. Her look is meditative. 'You're feeling stuck?'

I nod.

'Tell me about it.'

I tell her about sitting under the tree watching the light taken up into the leaves like syrup, watching the light and thinking about my death.

'The Verve is right,' I say. 'The drugs don't work.'

Helen smiles a little sadly. 'One step at a time. How are you managing with the drinking?'

'I'm drinking.'

'Any alcohol-free days?'

'Nope.'

I walk back outside, where Hana and Michael and Jack are sitting in the smoking alcove. Jack is the consumer consultant to the hospital and the Community Clinic. He's been a patient and is now a paid staff member. He organises meetings and workshops for patients and staff so that the hospital can learn from patients about what works and what doesn't. Hana has joined the team focusing on safety.

We sit together for a while in silence; companionable, smoke drifting to the sky. Michael smiles. His eyes are lit from deep inside, the brown penetrates. I walk home and take a couple of lorazepams. Rose is leaning over Henry as he stands by the sink. She washes his hands with bitter orange and bergamot, lathers fingers and palms and the backs of his hands where veins slide blue under the skin back toward the heart.

Such grace says Rose. They hold hands and the soapy water runs over their fine joints and away. In the night I open the bottle of yellow lorazepam and the bottle of blue alprazolam. The tablets are scored down the centre and powdery opaque; they sit like small circles of desire in my palm. The night air is tender, unruffled. The trees' leaves are backlit through the moon. I take the lorazepam and the alprazolam without water. Addiction to benzos is an insidious thing. The trick is to find someone who will prescribe it and then someone else who will prescribe it so that one can live on double the amount any one prescription provides. I am not mainlining – yet.

10

Absurdly, given my mental state, I apply for a job as a medical writer for an independent company in the city. I wonder if medical writing might be a way to combine knowledge (medicine) and passion (literature). I wear a new suit to the series of interviews, I have clean fingernails and a new haircut and I only drink a third of a bottle of whisky the night before.

The interviewers are nice. During the interviews I summon every atom of energy to ignore the people in my head, to walk into the room with a straight back, to shake hands and smile, to remember the interviewers' names and make a warm-but-not-too-intense kind of eye contact, to consider their questions carefully and to answer calmly, but with precision. I am acting in a play. I am assuming a character I wish was me – articulate and responsive and measured.

The new job is four days a week, writing articles for GPs in the core areas of general practice: ischaemic heart disease, asthma, diabetes, depression, hypertension, common infections in children, soft tissue injuries, arthritis. The other members of the 'team' are keenly self-sufficient and not particularly welcoming. I'm given a desk and a computer and I'm told to write an article on new drugs for congestive cardiac failure. There's a list of cardiologists and pharmacologists with whom I have to consult. My desk looks out onto the front of a BDSM house (bondage, discipline, sadomasochism). Occasionally one of the Mistresses comes out for a smoke dressed in a black shiny catsuit complete with tail and lace-up boots climbing her thighs.

The espresso machine confounds me. When I finally manage to make a cup of coffee my hands shake so much from the lithium that half of it spills as I walk back to my desk. The people in my head interject while I read journal articles—

spasm spam ride the blue train colitis mastitis arthritis red reel

Mornings I catch the train to work. There are other people on the train. Many of them. I'm afraid of their eyes. Carriage doors leer open, are disembowelled of people. Mobile phones ring and make me jump. Sometimes I can't find a space with enough air in it: there are bodies pressing, pressing, smelling of cigarettes and burnt cheese and blood and body odour. Bodies wriggling and scratching – the movement of flesh.

touch him touch her SCREAM

I stay very still, lines of sweat run down the back of my legs.

Once the sun is low enough in the sky after work I walk to the local pub. Candles along the bar and on the tables provide the only light, candles cosseted inside frosted glass so that the light is soft and foggy. The tables and chairs and floor and ceiling are old wood stained dark. It is warm. There are velvet curtains and few patrons, no racehorse or footballer photographs in gilt frames and no particular dress code. People sink into the couches. I unzip my coat and stretch out. I may stay here forever in this cocooning light, with whisky and black coffee, my scruffy notebooks and the sprung rhythm of GM Hopkins.

'Gin and tonic?' repeats the bar woman to someone with his back to me. 'Oh hell yeah, full of vitamins,' and they both laugh.

Dolly Parton is singing 'Jolene'. Jolene, please . . .

Easter. Though not of the Christian faith, Jesus' sort-of-suicide is fascinating and I carry around a quiet sadness – not about his death in particular but about Death and Grief. To find some spiritual space I book the cats into a cattery and pack the tent and camera and food and drive up to the Alpine National Park in northeastern Victoria.

My father taught me about photography when I was quite young. He had a Nikon SLR. Before I was born he worked in the ABC television studios so he knew all about light and perspective.

'Don't just snap away,' he'd say. 'Take your time. Think about your foreground. How can you make the photograph appear 3-dimensional?'

I love trying out new angles, changing the ISO or filter, lying flat on my back looking up the trunk of a tree, crouching in a corner, or waiting for thirty minutes till the light changes in the rain for that one shot when the pink sun bloodies rain drops and makes them live.

There's a car park off the Bogong High Plains Road from which I begin walking. This is the traditional country of the Bidawal people, the Dhudhuroa, Gunai-Kurnai and Nindi-Ngudjam Ngarigu Monero people. For thousands of years, other community groups joined them on the highest peaks in summer for corroborees and trade and to catch the nutrient-rich Bogong Moths. I love this land, but it is not my land. I trespass. I try to walk gently across the alpine grass plains, in between bunches of snow gums. Here, time is measured in sunlight and the autumn wind breath and the moon in the corner, thinned to a thread.

Once the endglow of the sun lowers itself below the horizon one must lie on the earth and look up. Eyes take about thirty minutes to dark-adapt. Pupils dilate. Rods and cones (photoreceptors) in the retina adjust sensitivity. Breathe in from the diaphragm, lungs to veins to arteries to heart and here they are, as they always are, and there are more of them than I'll ever have the ability to count and the longer I look – awe. Then dizziness like losing gravity, losing a sense of what is up and what is down. Some of them appear to coalesce into a kind of fine lace and some appear to be winking blue and some are occasionally but not always winking red and some yellow and some the whitest white. Mine one tiny view of the piebald vastness.

Back home, I go with Lara, who is beginning her training in pathology, to see *21 Grams*, a film about grief. The title refers to the amount of mass said to escape the body at the moment of death, the supposed weight of the soul. I take hold of the character played by Benicio del Toro, lost in grief after running over a father and his children in a truck. I understand his desperate need to atone for being alive. I have a desperate need to atone for being alive. After the film ends we have lunch, and then I catch a tram home via a hardware store where I buy a bottle of 32 per cent hydrochloric acid.

your duty is hell you know it we know it we are watching we are you sickbitch do it do it

I look at the body, the lump of flesh, fat and wavery and hirsute. Jeff Buckley is singing. I sit down on the floor in the hallway, smoke a cigarette, slop some bitter coffee.

flesh is hell flesh is hell flesh is hell flesh is hell we know we are watching now we are you bitch do it

Pour acid into a bowl, soak a towel in the acid and wrap it around the lower half of the right leg. I do it slowly. The pain is not immediate; there is a small lull in which silence stretches through my head on wings. The people in my head howl. Then a prickling, radiant heat envelops the leg all the way to the groin. I rock back and forth, eyes closed, head locked. I atone for Benicio del Toro, I atone. I lie on my side on the floorboards and my fat grey cat curls up under my chin. Her breath, her rhythmical breath falls on my lips.

How does one atone? It is partly the pain and partly the damage done that matters.

In the morning the leg is mottled pink and red with blisters and large patches of dried grey tissue that indicate third degree burns. I pull my pants over the mess and go to work as usual. First we have an all-department refresher in biostatistics to assist with our assessing of journal articles: hypothesis testing using p-values, confidence intervals, meta-analyses, quantitative versus qualitative research. I sit and listen with my forearms clasped under my right leg so that I don't have to put my right foot on the floor. After the meeting we stretch and yawn and make coffee.

'Good weekend?' I ask Tara, one of my colleagues.

'Oh great,' she says. 'We bought a pram that converts into about fifteen other things. Dan's obsessed with it.' Tara's six months pregnant with twins, so her belly looks more like eight months. She's switched from exhausted to glowing to exhausted to somehow rather serene.

'Excellent,' I say and smile. I've got all my weight on one leg, holding the wall.

'How was yours?' Tara asks.

'Went to see this amazing film.'

'Oh yeah? What was it?'

'*21 Grams.*'

'With Sean Penn? I know someone who saw that and said it was a bit, you know, blah blah blah. Awful script, I think he said. Did you like it?' She looks at her watch. 'Shit, sorry, teleconference. Catch up later?'

'Sure.' I walk back to my desk carefully. I've got a deadline in two days for an article on community-acquired pneumonia.

sick sick sickbitch hahaha

I ring a respiratory physician to get a second opinion about some of the recommended medications in the article. His secretary pages him and he rings back and we chat for awhile and I thank him and finish the article and email it to my boss for his opinion and I don't leave my desk all day because walking is too painful. I say I've brought lunch from home, thank you anyway, and leave my bladder to fill and fill until everyone has left for the evening and I half-creep half-limp to the bathroom and then to the train.

Over the week the patches of grey enlarge like moss over tiles. I'm careful to wear opaque stockings. When the pain prevents sleep, I visit Jenny, my GP, who takes a look and writes a referral to the local emergency department. In the waiting room are an old Greek couple, some young men from Africa and a man lying on his back on the floor in a corner. The triage nurse takes me straight through to a cubicle. Next door someone is having a catheter inserted, I can hear him moaning.

Vanessa, the nurse, sets up an IV line. 'I think you'll be admitted,' she says. 'Is there anyone I can call?'

'No thanks.' She gives me a starchy white gown, open at the back. I wait several hours, staring at the nylon curtains; pale blue with a thin white stripe. I follow the stripe with my eyes updownupdown. The plastics registrar examines the leg. He's young and efficient in his clean white coat, and he looks at my leg but not at my face.

'It probably needs surgical debridement and a split-skin graft. I'll go and get your file.' He returns some time later. 'I'm not prepared to give you the surgery.'

'Why not?' I ask.

'Because this is deliberate self harm, not an accident.'

My insides sink down below the bed. The registrar shuffles through my file.

'Would you have the surgery, if you were in my position, with this injury?' I ask.

'Of course.'

'Are you discriminating against me on account of mental illness?'

'It's not cost effective for the hospital because you have a history of self-harm. In the same way we discriminate against smokers who need lung transplants.' He walks away.

sick sick sickbitch sick sick sickbitch sick aahhaha

Vanessa looks surprised. 'I'm sorry,' she says. 'Would you like to make a complaint?'

Still with my insides sunk down below my feet, I smile, 'No bloody point.' Anyway, the registrar is probably right. I'm not cost effective. After she leaves, I get off the bed; put my clothes back on and slide the IV needle out of my arm. Walk out into the night.

It is Friday evening. Zoë and I are at the Northcote Social Club to see an Adelaide band called Fruit. Zoë and I found each other at a personal development course in St Kilda five years ago. Somehow we survived the barely controlled rooms of people shouting and crying and bashing pillows. We both knew depression and we were looking for a way through. Not a way out necessarily, but insight into the why of it. If we understood that, maybe we could stop it. Maybe we could become strong enough to just stop it – make it go away, make it never come back.

Zoë is clever, shy, beautiful. Cornflower blue eyes, perfect skin. But much more than that, in her eyes and smile, is depth. The depth is, I think, part intellect and part warmth and part knowledge of suffering. We click without effort, occasionally opening our naked selves; finding connection and then the relief that we're not so alone.

Still, I'm too scared to ask the people I love for help. Tonight the acoustic guitar and harmonising voices wash over me like warm honey and I'm sweating and shivering and swaying with the music. I try to dance on one leg; the pain in the other is intense and unrelenting. Lymph nodes behind my knee and deep in my groin are swollen and tender, sweat runs down my back and pools in my underwear. The leg itself is pink as salmon. After the concert I assure Zoë that I'm 'fine, really, don't worry,' and instead of asking her to come with me, I drive alone to the nearest Emergency Department.

The surgical registrar calls the plastics registrar who decides on emergency surgery. I'm wheeled off to theatre after a dose of morphine and a dose of antibiotics. The anaesthetics registrar explains the procedure for the anaesthetic but I'm too drowsy to hear her. I wake up with someone rubbing my sternum.

'Breathe Kate,' I nod comprehension. 'Your oxygen sats are too low.' I nod again and breathe. Up in the ward I'm given another dose of morphine and I float up to the ceiling from where I look down on the body as it lies in the bed. The ceiling light is very white.

rouge rough fat arse red fucking lunatic

Outside I can see the nebulous blobs of light where cars are whisking by in the rain and the night, but it is quiet in here. A nurse quietly checks my blood pressure and pulse and takes my temperature. I try to sleep. Rose and Henry lie beside me, their clothes, velvet and linen, smoothed out on the bed. They start to sing, a low, graceful cadence.

chords flow over our brow, deep in ink and pure silk, swim beneath composure, open outward, lotus-like, enter us and refract, blur, cover white walls, move in our white skin

A skin graft is a sliver of skin shaved from a large area like the thigh and transplanted to the area of injury after the debridement of damaged tissue. New blood vessels begin growing from the recipient area into the transplanted skin within 36 hours. My skin grafts look like punched out circles of the brightest red, gel-like and impossibly fragile. I ring work and tell them I've had 'surgery.' I imagine they'll think it's the gynaecological kind. My parents visit and bring me flowers; we don't talk about the reason for the wounds, but I appreciate their quiet support. I tell ward staff that the whole thing was an accident, that I dropped the bottle of hydrochloric acid on my foot. They ask me every morning if I would like to 'speak to someone'.

I wait in the light from the window in the day and I wait in the light from the corridor at night for healing. The people in my head are quieter here but there are still cameras in the air conditioning vents and at the back of the television. Leering. I'm embarrassed to use the bedpan.

The hospital chaplain asks if he can sit and talk with me awhile.

I shift in the bed so I can face him.

'How are you?' he asks.

'Fine. Thank you. Kind of . . . fine. Well. Ah.'

The chaplain's expression is mild, like warm milk. Suddenly, unexpectedly, I wish I could embrace someone. Not the chaplain necessarily, but someone. A fine, beautiful embrace.

'How is it, being here in hospital?' he asks.

Slowly. To hold . . . to give . . . and to hold.

'Yes. Sorry,' I say. 'Pardon?'

'How is it, being here in hospital?'

rough fat arse red fucking lunatic

They stick back in like knives. I flinch. Rearrange the blankets.

'Well. A lot of things . . . I get so confused. And. It's like having stumbled out of the normal stream of life.'

'It is okay to have some time out.'

I nod.

'Who is at home with you?'

'Home alone.' I try not to sound too pathetic.

'Friends?'

'Yes. I love them.'

'Friends are a blessing.'

'Yes.'

'Peace be with you.'

'And also with you.'

The clouds move swiftly past my window, dark grey on light grey on dark grey, forming shapes like mountains in the air. It rains. There is beauty in the way sunlight streams through a gap in the clouds, the smallest glimpse of heaven. I listen to the sound of rain on the roof and sleep.

The plastics registrar sends me home in the morning with a plaster cast on my leg and a pair of crutches. Home is books and music, Rose and Henry, a safe place, a sanctuary. Home is also benzos and booze.

kill fucking ugly useless lump of flesh useless unless keep the fires burning burn and sway get your head read all red underneath flesh

I sit in an armchair with a cat on my lap and think about this. I try to breathe. I find some Jim Beam in the cupboard under the sink and pour half a glass and drink it, letting my throat and gullet burn. Soon enough I'm being washed in warm water, swung gently from side to side as in a low tide, my head just above the edges of the waves. While drunk I have a frank conversation with Zoë on the phone about alcohol and about suicide. We touch on ownership, abandonment, integrity, grief, hope, meds and therapy. We touch on death and what it means to still be alive in spite of everything. We reminisce, we laugh. I agree to think about finding a therapist, and I also decide to make a formal complaint to the Patient Advocate at the hospital where I was refused treatment. In part I say, '. . . Surely you will agree that this is a serious breach of care and blatant discrimination on the part of Dr X. Further it demonstrates his inexcusable ignorance of the nature of acute mental illness, and the possible repercussions for patients, like myself, who are then left to manage on their own. The consequences for me may well have included non-healing of the wounds, serious localised infection and septicaemia.'

I lie in bed and wonder about sleep; I keep counsel with the night. Rose and Henry lie together holding hands, the cool breeze sliding in between their fingers, titillating. Thoughts zig zag and merge into dreams. This is what it is to be alone, to be without the touch of another human being, a quiescent soul. I put on Schubert's String Quartet in D Minor: *Death and the Maiden*. The *andante con moto* movement swells purely and falls and rises again. I take a lorazepam. The night stretches out in the strange quiet and later abuts the light as it becomes inch by inch brighter. My big cat stretches, curls his big feet inward, lengthens them towards the ceiling, sighs and goes back to sleep.

II

At the Community Clinic, Jim says I should stay off the venlafaxine. Michael is clearly agitated, pacing and talking to himself, his cap pulled down low. I leave him alone. Rachel and Hana are playing pool.

'You deserve to win,' says Hana.

'These balls are hypnotic,' says Rachel.

'You can't take them home,' says Hana.

'I want to put them in my garden. I could make a sculpture, a bird or a frog.'

'Go on then.'

Rachel arranges the balls on the table into a bird with red wings and a yellow beak and blue feet.

'That's a serious bird,' I say.

'I was a graphic designer in another life,' she says. 'Before the DSP vortex.'

'The what?'

'Disability Support Pension. Otherwise known as – life outside life.'

I nod. Hana nods.

Helen and I discuss psychotherapy. She gives me the business card of a private psychiatrist in Richmond, Paul L. 'He has a good reputation,' she says. I stare at her and pocket the card.

Paul's clinic is an old double storey home complete with wrought iron lace work and a fountain in the front. The stairs creak under my crutches. Despite the size of the building, his room is pokey, painted sandy brown and without a window. He has M.C. Escher on all four of his walls – things metamorphosing and reappearing, birds in disguise, fish being liberated from diamonds and squares. I leave after fifty minutes. All I remember about the session are the birds and fish and the bill for $110 and Paul's eyebrows that are so pale his forehead goes on forever.

A week later Paul suggests I see him in his own home in the inner east, where he does evening appointments. His home is a Victorian terrace, there are several fat cats sitting on the porch. He ushers me into a room with a bookshelf running floor to ceiling and a chaise lounge up against one wall.

'Do you like Leonard Cohen?' he asks. 'I think you'd like his poetry – start with *Stranger Music*.'

'I'll note it down,' I say.

'How do you feel about hypnotherapy?'

'Oh God no.'

'It could be very helpful – for you.'

He gets up from his chair in the corner and sits down next to me on the lounge, less than a hands-breadth away, I can feel his warmth.

'It's perfectly safe,' he holds his arms out wide and then lets one of his hands browse my knee as it comes back down, a fleeting touch. I shiver, then freeze. My mouth moves but everything else is stuck shut. The people in my head roar.

'I'll think about it.' I try to say it normally, he is so close, my lungs hurt, he is so close, I want to get off the lounge, my legs fail me.

'Good, you have a think about it,' he says, smooths down his pants and stands up. 'See you next week.' I get to my feet by swivelling around and pushing myself up with my arms. I walk like I do

Somewhere between caricature & erotisism Andre Kertesz's art called 'Distortion.'

Unsure how long I can maintain the calm. Head & heart full of the boiling, biting, angry deamons. They sit ready with watchful eyes, they pounce on every move, every expression, the very heartbeat & the feel of air. They whip & beat, tease, seize hold of my soul and run with its bloodied shreds in their teeth. They are unaware of the word 'cease'. They do not tire and for some reason they do not die. Full of morning mourning. I cannot eat or sleep.

Memory

when I'm drunk, watching my feet, thinking about the right place to put them down, and recommence breathing in my car. There's sweat and urine in my pants.

One day I leave work early and go for a walk in the park near my block of flats. I'm limping along without crutches, without the plaster cast that is lying alone on my living room floor. In the park a young boy is playing football with his father. He kicks the ball high into the air right into the blue of the sky; it lands a few feet in front of him which he finds tremendously funny. His father chases him to the ball, both of them running and laughing, then they roll over and over, the freshly mown grass covering their clothes like fur.

I sit down on the edge of the oval with my notebooks and some Octavio Paz to read and write and think. The inner world, the heart of things, where truths lie mired by the inconstant voices of reason and unreason, are doubly mired by the people living in my head – the bitter ones, the sarcastic ones, the demons, between whom there is an ever-evolving dance that allows me little rest. I'm not managing. I need help, but I don't know how to find the right help. In the sky cirrus clouds are forming a long, fibrous mare's tail, signalling an approaching storm. I wonder how soft they are. The sky in between is a perfect blue.

Having always respected the discipline and art of psychology, I heave the Yellow Pages onto my bed and look up 'psychologist'. There are hundreds listed. I find one whose practice is nearby – Jane. It takes me several days to gather the courage to call her. In the meantime I take benzos and supplement with alcohol to drown the internal cacophony.

pierce piece bit ride the horse sunlit shit keep floating drown drown yourself gutter black

Jane asks me why I want to see a psychologist. I tell her about the depression. The day-in-day-out grind that is living with depression. I tell her I've suffered bouts of it lasting months since I was sixteen and that I don't understand why. And I tell her that I don't trust psychiatrists. She listens. We agree to an initial session in a week.

Despite the heat I wear a long skirt, stockings, a jumper and a grey overcoat made of merino wool. My hands are shaking. I take the tram and then walk to Jane's office, outside of which I stand for a considerable period of time. Once inside I sit in the waiting room with *Death in Venice* by Thomas Mann. It is beautiful writing, in parts it sings. It is also terribly serious, a little oppressive and a little depressing. On the wall is a Rene Magritte print *The Empire of Lights II*, a tantalising scene of a house in the evening with a day-lit blue sky and clouds overhead. The dark and light of the mind? A representation of the conscious and the unconscious?

'Come on in, Kate,' says Jane.

'Thank you.' I wrap the overcoat around me tightly.

keep the fires burning you are dead kill her you are dead the trees are shivering

The room is rectangular with windows down one long side letting the light in. There are two black lounge chairs set almost opposite one another on an Afghani rug. One wall is a bookshelf half full of books and the other a fireplace with glass ornaments and a black and white photo of the Lubavitcher Rebbe on the mantelpiece. I sit down.

'Tell me about yourself.'

My legs are shaking and my hands are shaking and my voice comes out wavery and thin like the end of a whistle. I can't breathe with the depth of her eyes across the room.

'Well . . . I'm twenty-eight, mostly ordinary. Normal childhood and all that, um, I'm an only child. Grew up on a farm. Both parents alive and well. I live on my own. No children because I'm afraid I'd be a dreadful parent. I work and . . . I'm crazy about wilderness and all kinds of music and feline personalities and I'm a peacenik or a wanker whichever way you choose to look at it. That's it really. Oh, and I hate – I mean hate as in wish to kill – pretty much everything about me. I guess you should know that.'

We agree to two more introductory sessions. I walk home with the sunshine at my feet and I walk through part of my shadow, and keep walking past the green grocers with their piles of oranges and spring onions and potatoes, past the clothing shops and the boys busking with flute and violin outside the newsagency, past the bottle shop. I turn the corner and walk by the tram tracks and have trouble looking up into the sun.

the glare will blind you bind you raw we'll bury you

Rose and Henry are home. I take a couple of lorazepams, little yellow suns.

touch me says Rose. Henry runs the back of his hand from the very top of her head over her cheek, her neck, her breasts. Soft as a moth's wing, a mere breath. Rose shivers. I curl up with a scotch and soda and with *Midnight's Children*, and am immediately immersed in Kashmir pre-partition. The people in my head can hardly get a word in, they shuffle and mumble on the outskirts of consciousness. I hit my head, hard, to keep them in their place.

The sky outside has splotches of red where the clouds meet the blue; my eyes feel raw. I take another yes-I-love-you benzo and lie down to await its effect: the drowsing dreaminess, the gentle half-sleep. I watch the clock tick tick and breathe on every alternate stroke. Rose and Henry watch me from the corner of the room. I slide, the room quietens.

On the footpath of Fitzroy Street on a Saturday afternoon a man sits with a llama tied up by his side. The llama looks mildly surprised. Someone is busking with a didgeridoo. It is very warm, the concrete shimmers whitely, the asphalt shimmers blackly. Couples walk by with babies, their prams shrouded. An enormous black dog hops along on three legs. I wonder if everyone is questioning what it is to be alive on this particular day at this particular time. I am amazed by it. Two bikers sit at the next table. Heads shaved, reflective sunglasses, beards, earrings – gold and silver hoops, leather jackets, black jeans, leather boots. It is disconcerting not to see their eyes.

Down on the beach the waves break their salty stories over the shore, sea gulls dance on gusts of wind and there are people kite-surfing out in deeper water. I sit on the low concrete wall and dangle my feet in sand that is coarse and warm and yellow. The sand tickles between my toes. I keep my normal face on – the face that says I am-just-another-young-woman-enjoying-the-beach-on-the-weekend, perhaps waiting for her boyfriend or her husband to bring ice cream and love.

12

A month passes in which I visit Jane several times and we talk about depression – beginning at age fifteen and extending episodically through the later years of school and all of university, through family holidays and birthdays and the weddings of friends.

'You went to uni?' she asks.

'Yes.'

'What did you study?'

'Medicine.'

'Really?'

'Graduated with honours. In between hospitalisations.'

'How did you manage to pass your exams?' she asks.

'Bursts of extreme concentration. Some days I'd study for twelve hours straight. Other days I didn't get out of bed.'

'How about school?'

'It wasn't ever what I'd call serious depression at school. But I think it was more extreme than the normal teenage emotional rollercoaster. When I was seventeen I knew, I mean I *really* knew, that I could go on living for a couple more years at most. I was exhausted. Turing up to school every day and trying to appear normal when inside . . . I was a witch or a banshee or I was dead and rotting or I was just plain ridiculous depending on the day. It was exhausting.'

'So are you practicing medicine?'

'I can't, well I mean I wouldn't – I mean if something happened, if I made a mistake because I was unwell, I'd never forgive myself.'

'All that training!' she says.

we're killing you bitch ahhaha on the ground

I look at her hard. 'Yes.'

'Did you want to work in a hospital or general practice?'

'Neither. I've always wanted to be a forensic physician.'

'Cutting up dead bodies?'

'That's a forensic pathologist. I mean someone who takes care of women and men after a sexual assault and sees people who have been injured in prison or in police custody and—'

'That sounds tough.'

'Some days. I spent time at the Institute for Forensic Medicine as a student. It didn't matter to me what people had done or were accused of doing, and it wasn't all violence-related. We also assessed whether people were okay to be interviewed or give evidence or stand for trial and we gave medical advice to police and the courts. Every single day was fascinating. It was . . . I think it was my calling, if such a thing exists.'

'Yes?'

'Not in a religious sense. It just felt right.'

'But you're not doing that now?'

'No. Couldn't do any of the preliminary hospital training. Kept getting sick.'

'Is that disappointing?'

'No, no,' I say. 'Could be worse.'

No, no. Could be a lot worse, could be a garbo or something, could be unemployed, could be dead, it's fine, fine really, all that studying just in time for one's mind to fail, to haul oneself back up and then it fails again . . . and again.

'What do you do now?'

'Working as a medical writer.'

'What do you write about?'

'Right now we're developing an update for GPs on the treatment of acute leukaemia.'

'How's you concentration at work?'

I laugh.

Jane raises her eyebrows. 'That's funny?'

you are blind dead dead whine red ha ha

'Hah. I mean, no. No. But—'

ha ha ha ha blind dead blind

'I . . . have a nasty habit of . . . things get weirdly adulterated in here,' I tap my head. I smile. Then my eyes fill. Of their own accord. 'Um . . . juggling is required. Severe focus. Attention to multiple inputs of data at the same time.'

'Oh?'

'Like you are listening to the radio through one ear and the television through the other.'

'Mmm. Do you ever get high – I mean your mood?'

I grin, mouthandeyes, and uncross my legs, leaving my knees open. 'Sometimes it's like being on speed and Es together, without the come-down.'

'Does it ever go too far?'

'Been known to.' I re-cross my legs. 'That's when I start chain-smoking. Once I thought I'd discovered a new dimension. You know, there's length, width and depth, and time – the fourth dimension. Well I found a fifth. So I thought.'

Jane has long black hair with a curious streak of light grey at the front that matches her eyes. Her voice is soft, measured, uncluttered, a little hypnotic.

'What's your earliest memory?' she asks.

Orange light, a curtain, the dark, no one there, just the orange light and the dark and silence like fog, endless orange light and the dark.

'About age seven. There was a deep frost, and the dogs made shining green footprints in the grass and the ice-crystals crackled under their feet.'

'What about before the age of seven?'

'Fog.'

'Fog?'

I think for a moment and nod. 'Fog.'

'Why are you wearing so many clothes?' Jane asks at the next session.

'Covers the ugliness up. I'd cover my face as well if I could.'

'Are you ugly, Kate?'

I stare at the floor, I don't blink, I don't move.

'Disgusting.' I say it so low it's almost a growl.

Jane sits still but I start to shake, first my hands and arms, then my legs, then my torso, not an epileptic seizure, more like someone with hypothermia. My teeth are chattering, my eyes are watering, I can't blink. Jane comes over to my chair and puts her hand on my shoulder but I shudder further and flinch, and she removes it.

'Can I do anything for you Kate?' she asks very quietly. I can't stop the shaking, it's as though an animal inside me is trying to get out. Sweat is running into my eyes and down my back and under my breasts. I keen. The people in my head scream.

Jane sits down and waits. After some minutes the shaking subsides. I blink. She gives me some tissues and I wipe my face and neck.

'Sorry,' I say.

'Has that happened before?' she asks.

'Yes,' I say, then I say, 'We never discuss the body.'

'We?'

I stare at her. 'Yes.'

'Who is "we"?'

I try to speak, but the people in my head gag me. They make me put my hands around my throat and exert pressure on my carotid arteries and my trachea. The room goes fuzzy. They start to wail and cajole—

rip yourself stab knife your heart stick it in

'Kate, can you hear me?'

I nod.

'You're perfectly okay here.'

I open my eyes.

'It's okay.'

bleed for this

The tram arrives

bleed for this

and I get on and

bleed for this

fall into one of the lumpy seats and cover my eyes with my palms. The chatter from the other passengers sounds like rain, except that it is also made up of colour – blues and oranges and violet; all falling from above and falling around me. If I put my arms out, palms up, the colours patter onto my skin and return to white. I step off the tram. My legs are still shaking and I look up through the dark

bleed for this

and there's a halo around the full moon – another (fainter) perfect circle.

My little flat has the pale smell of unburnt sandalwood incense. The cats uncurl and reach out with their front paws

you will bleed for this

and mrrrrl and lift their furry heads. Their eyes are finer than glass. I feed them and sort through the pile of CDs on the floor in the living room and here is Boccherini's cello concerto. It is his Concerto no. 9, in B-flat Major.

bleed for this bleeeed

'Number nine in B flat major,' I say loudly to drown them. 'Number nine in B flat major number nine in B flat major.'

The adagio is a simple, slow melody until a solo cello stretches beyond the orchestra – holding a note that little bit longer, like a story within a story or the deepest insides of a flower. It settles me. I think I'll be okay. 'Number nine in B flat major.'

But in the morning I can't face work.

bleed for this bleed you YOU

I'm up on time and clothed appropriately and

bleed for this we will make you bleed for this

then I sink down into the couch with my back straight, hands folded, feet neatly together on the floor and I don't move, I don't move while the clock's hands proceed from eight to nine to ten – my body is somehow locked up. Eventually I ring to

bleed for this

apologise and the guilt seeps in.

The corner of Carlisle and Chapel is a drop in centre for folk with psychiatric illness. It provides meals and activities and support. I sit out the front on the side of the road, never having mustered the courage to go inside. Coming towards me is an oldish woman pulling a cart with three wheels and inside the cart is a little white dog with eyes like mercury.

'Shantih, Shantih, Shantih,' she sings in time with her feet. The dog smiles right back at her. His fur and her hair mirror one another. I go into a cafe and the coffee comes with an extra shot and a heart etched into its creamy surface. I turn it around to drink left-handed and the heart is now an onion.

bleed for this we will make you you will bleeeeeeed for this

On the way home I go into the 7-Eleven and buy a pack of Winfield Blues and a cigarette lighter and at home I light a cigarette.

bleed haha

I keep one end in my mouth, sit on the floor in half-lotus, hold the other end, the lit end, against the skin of the middle of my calf. I inhale and exhale. The cigarette flares and dies. I re-light it. The skin blushes pink then red then grey. It is raining. Rain drops fall and pool on leaves and fall again to the ground. The air is musty with the day's heat, the room full of smoke and the people in my head finally stop shouting.

Later I put on Elgar's Cello Concerto in E Minor. It is music that reaches into the depths of things, like light into water. The sound of the cello is exquisite and absolute but by accident I brush against my leg and a shiver of pain runs up into my groin.

To my next appointment with Jane, I wear a long skirt over jeans and long black boots and an overcoat, scarf and beanie. My knees are wool.

'How have you been?' Jane asks.

I shrug, 'Comme ci comme ça, aval kacha ha'chayim.'

'What do you mean in English?'

'Terrified.'

'Of . . .?'

sssssss vile we will make you we have you WE ARE YOU die

I flinch.

'Can you tell me what you are terrified of?' Jane asks, very quietly.

I don't blink for a long time and then the clock clicks on Jane's desk and the sound fills my ears and reverberates there; little sound waves piling in upon themselves, clickclickclick. I tap the side of my head hard and stretch and smile.

'Shit,' I say.

'I'm . . . strangled,' I say. 'Sorry.'

The burn inevitably gets infected. My ankle swells so that socks leave detailed patterns on my skin, dips and ridges and furrows. It smells slightly rotten; to compensate I spray a lot of green-tea perfume and rub orange oil over my clothes. In the evenings I take a lorazepam and a couple of phenergans and go to bed and dream of being shot in the head.

At the next session, Jane notices that I can't bend my right knee properly, and I explain.

'Is it painful?' she asks.

'Yes.'

'You remind me of the way Hitler treated the Jews,' she says, leaning forward in her chair. I choke on some saliva. The air leaves my lungs. I stare at her for a moment then quietly gather my bag and books and walk out. I walk fast down the road while the people in my head scream and I narrowly avoid an oncoming car, its horn blares, I drop my pile of books and scrabble on the ground in the middle of the road with my squelchy shoe and sweaty palms and runny nose.

At home I light some incense and watch smoke rise cylindrically to the roof. I screw the body up tight and shove my mind into the farthest corner of my brain with Jack Daniels. But the fact remains. Jane has confirmed it. There is something intrinsically wrong with me, something rotten. Something analogous to Hitler.

13

On my day off work Helen meets me in the hallway of the Community Clinic and we walk together to her office.

'I feel sick,' I tell her. 'Jane is Jewish. Anyone can make a comment about Hitler. But a comment from someone whose family may have been murdered in the Holocaust carries so much more weight. And meaning. It's an enormous, awful analogy. It's so black and awful. I don't think I can go back.'

Helen puts her head on one side and sighs.

'How is your leg?' she asks.

'Fine,' I say.

'Kate, it smells. Are you cleaning it?'

'No.'

'I'm going to ask CATT to come and see you in the evening.'

The Crisis Assessment and Treatment Team (CATT) is a part of every public hospital psych department. The team is responsible for assessing people in the community who may need admission to hospital because they are in the acute phase of a psychiatric illness or are exhibiting symptoms that may be the result of a psychiatric illness. Symptoms could include hallucinations, delusions, persistent thoughts of suicide or homicide or other symptoms of mania, depression, psychosis and severe anxiety that place the person at risk of harm to themselves or others.

Two psych nurses, members of CATT, come around in the early evening. The evening itself is pure and clear. I sit cross-legged on the floor.

'Do you understand why we're here?' one asks.

'Well I think so, but really, there's no need, I'm perfectly alright, my brain's just a bit tight.'

scream a black dream

'How is your leg?'

'Fine.'

'What did you do to it?'

'Burnt it.'

'Can we have a look?' They lean forward. I pull at my sock; it's stuck to the wound so I peel it away slowly.

shhhhhhh bitch

'You need to get that cleaned up. And you need antibiotics.'

'No,' I say.

'Why not?'

'No.'

'You'll lose your leg or the infection will spread into your bloodstream. Do you want to die Kate?'

'I do.'

'Why?'

'I deserve it. It's my fate.'

'What medication are you on?'

'Lithium.'

'Will you let us clean up your leg?' I don't say anything. 'Otherwise we will have to take you to hospital.' I bang my hands on the floor, look at the walls, the ceiling. There's a crack in the corner of the ceiling where it meets the wall, black and sudden. The people in my head hiss and laugh—

we're killing you

'I don't know what to do,' I whisper.

'How about we start by cleaning the wound?'

I sit there on the floor amongst the mess of flesh with my heart hammering out an irregular beat and my head full of bile and the acute taste of venom.

touch us put your hands around usssss

I put my hands around my throat. There is sweat there, in the folds of skin that feel soft and wet as dough and are equally malleable. I look into the eyes of the members of the CAT team. Green eyes, brown eyes, liquid and light.

dead already

'I'm dead already,' I whisper.

'No, you're not. We can help you.' I look up at them from the depths of a well, depths that have swallowed earth and sky.

you deserve this

'I deserve this,' I say.

'Kate, you are not thinking clearly. Now we need to clean up your leg and get you some antibiotics. We would like you to come with us.'

'Okay,' I say, with my hands around my throat. 'Okay.'

We walk down the stairs and out to the CAT team car. It is a white Toyota, small and functional, just the right size for taking people off to hospital. I sit in the back with my oversize bag of books and the little rivulets of serous fluid running into my shoes.

The Emergency Department is all bright lights and people moving fast. A man lies on a trolley in the corridor by the waiting room with eyes yellow as a cat's. I am left to wait in the cubicle with the solid walls and the lockable, solid door. I wait for several hours. The members of the CAT team return. 'We'll get a doctor to come and look at your leg and then the psychiatric registrar on call will come and assess you.'

The desire to get up off the trolley that is narrow and cold and walk out into the night is compelling. Two security guards walk by in their grey uniforms with their mounds of keys, a nurse takes my blood pressure and pulse and temperature and brings me a warmed blanket and later a resident examines my leg and prescribes a stat dose of IV antibiotics and some oxycodone for pain relief. My mind is vacuous as a shell; equally made up of circles within circles of smooth, shining material that from the outside appear perfect but are rotten within.

'Are you feeling down or depressed for most of the day?' asks the psych registrar, sitting legs crossed neatly with sheer stockings and shiny high heels and a dress to match her eyes.

I nod slowly. 'Most days.'

'How are you sleeping?'

'A few hours a night.'

'What about concentration?'

'Terrible.'

'Are you hearing things that other people can't hear?'

'No.'

'Are you seeing things that other people can't see?'

'No.'

'Is the television or radio broadcasting special messages for you?'

'No.'

'Do you think that anyone is trying to harm you?'

'No.'

'Are you thinking about dying?'

'Yes.'

She looks surprised. I don't think she believes me. I stay overnight on the cold and narrow trolley in the room with the solid walls and am discharged in the early morning with a packet of antibiotics and a muddy-red heart. I go straight in to work, fumble with the espresso machine, smile brightly as people arrive to begin the day. The CAT team visit for a week to monitor the taking of the antibiotics as prescribed.

At the Community Clinic Helen and I talk about trying therapy again. I'm loath to enter into another relationship, to consider trust, to open my pale insides to someone new.

'I never thought I'd end up like this, Helen.' I say. 'Needing therapy. On medication. Not managing to be a normal adult. Not fucking managing.'

Helen raises her eyebrows. 'You can do this.'

I walk home with leaves gusting along at my feet. The Australian Psychological Society has a website with a 'find a psychologist' page. I select 'Depression' and 'Self Harm' as relevant categories and am furnished with a list of eight psychologists, each of whom has a detailed profile. Winsome works with cognitive-behavioural therapy (CBT), gestalt, humanistic and psychodynamic therapy. I like CBT and I like gestalt. Gestalt is a German word for form or shape. In English, it refers to a concept of wholeness. Gestalt therapy is a method of awareness of the individual's experience in the present moment. It is holistic; it emphasises personal responsibility and mind-body-culture relationships – all things I pound through life without considering. I ring Winsome and make an appointment, take a lorazepam and a bottle of Chivas Regal and curl up on the couch.

My diet consists of chocolate bars, alcohol and coffee. Occasionally I supplement with ice cream. I am enmeshed in Freud's oral stage of psychosexual development, stuck with a single erogenous zone – my mouth. Freud would say I am fixated.

The fruit and vegetable aisles in my local supermarket are a mystery. I am terrified of the supermarket. The lights are white hot and insistent, the isles bursting with shelf upon shelf of objects that pelt me with their colour and their words. It's hard to breathe. There is the hum of trolleys and air conditioning and people talking. The voice over makes me jump and once my legs start to shake I forget what I came to buy and leave with nothing but a pair of sweaty hands.

14

Winsome's office is upstairs, up a narrow little staircase that creaks. On the ground floor of her building is a natural therapies shop stocking strange herbs and books on iridology and homeopathy and pranic healing. I am suspicious of everything.

'Tell me why you're here,' Winsome says. I have my coat and my piles of notes and books. Winsome thinks there are only two of us in this consulting room, but she is wrong. I mumble something about blackness and despair, it is all they will allow, and then I look up at her and say, 'Sooner or later I'll end up like the poet Hart Crane and my friend John.'

'Oh?'

'Dead.'

Because after each episode of illness, I kept getting up and trying again and I never knew it could or would ever happen again and it did. It does. It keeps happening.

She looks at me with eyes that are kind and tired. We talk about my normal family and then about my childhood which was also normal, until things started to go wrong at sixteen.

'My mum and dad had a farm with hens and goats and cows and a horse and all sorts of fruit trees and acres of forest up the very back which I'd hide away in to think and to read. We lived there till I was about fourteen. I loved that farm. I was well there.'

'School?' she asks.

'All of us white, Anglo girls with very middle, middle class, white, Anglo backgrounds, all learning that Australia was discovered in 1789 but learning nothing that mattered about the traditional owners of the land. The school was a bit like a sheltered workshop, cocoon-like. I don't think we understood anything about real sickness or not having enough money, and we didn't ever mingle with the juxtaposition of cultures living an hour or so down the road. It's so sad to think about that. And embarrassing. But I had some great friends, beautiful, amazing friends. Still do. And my English teacher, Mrs Manton, saved my life back then. She showed me this other world: edgy theatre, modern art and literature. She was so generous. I think she kind of saw inside me and she didn't run from what she saw there. As a fifteen year-old, that meant more than anything.'

'What happened when you were sixteen?'

'It was strange. Although at the time I'm not sure I knew it was strange, which is itself strange. I'd always been a placid little lake and over a few months in 1990 I was overcome by a hurricane that never quite ever went away.'

Winsome's face mirrors compassion; it's there in her eyes so I know it's real, and it gives me courage.

'I had these fits of black rage and fits of melancholy that went on for days and during both I thought seriously about dying. Some of the time I was terrified, some of the time I was okay and some of the time I was . . . kind of smug.'

Winsome doesn't say anything for a moment. Then she asks quietly, 'Smug?'

'Yeah, because . . . this is weird, I know, but for a year or so when I was about seventeen, I thought I was the only one who knew that *all* of us were being followed and monitored and periodically fiddled with.'

'Fiddled with?'

'Tinkered with, like electronic toys, and impregnated while we slept. Or if we didn't sleep, we were drugged. As part of The Great Experiment.'

'Can you tell me more about that?'

Winsome has gently peeled back a layer, several layers, without me realising it and suddenly I'm aware of my awful nakedness. 'No. That's all there is.'

'Are you okay, Kate?' she asks. She sits still while I gather myself up.

'Sure. Fine. See you next week, Winsome. Thanks.'

When I walk back down the stairs and out into the sunlight my knees hardly bend.

Hana is not at the Community Clinic in the morning, nor the following week or the one after or the one after that. Hana with her beautiful voice and yellow tights. Her web page of music and social commentary and poetry has vanished into the cyber-ether. I don't know where she lives. Staff of course, won't give client information to other clients. I wander around the city at night, buy a drink, sit on the steps of Flinders Street Station with the goths and the punks and a few homeless folk, put my hands under my chin and wrap my coat around me, let the night go by. The police appear out of their mirrored compound and start talking to people on the steps, encouraging us to move on. I walk over to McDonald's for a coffee and stand on the sidewalk of Swanston Street, feeling the air, feeling the coffee raw in my mouth. My heart hurts. My stupid heart hurts.

'What do you do for fun?' Winsome asks one evening. She has big windows that run down the long side of the room and let in the last of the light. I look at her. Winsome is petite in the French sense: short in stature, slender, delicate feet and hands, stylish – in here my shabbiness sours.

'Fun?' I say.

'Yes.'

The silence expands.

I smile then and keep smiling and fold my hands together tight tight. It is a bittersweet feeling, like watching couples holding hands. The wonder of it. That touch. The wonder of fun.

When I leave her office I catch a tram to St Kilda, to the Voodoo Ink tattooing studio on Carlisle Street. I have a couple of cans of rum and coke along the way.

'What can we do for ya?' asks Luis, the tattoo artist.

'I'd like an owl,' I say. 'On my ankle.' Luis gets out some books on birds – eagles and toucans and bowerbirds and emus. We choose a black-and-white barn owl. Luis traces the outline onto paper. The owl stands about 10 centimetres tall. Luis draws in a tree branch and then goes to mix up the ink; grey and black. He gets me to sit in the old leather chair with my leg out straight. He says nothing about the scars.

A tattoo machine deposits ink into the dermis via four or five needles that press into the skin 80–150 times a second. It feels like a thousand tiny insect bites. I watch the slow creation of art on my skin; a body, a face, a pair of wings. Gracile and clear. I offer Luis some rum and coke. He laughs. 'No thanks, love. I'll get into trouble.'

When the tattoo is finished there's a raised red reaction around the edges of the inked skin. It's mildly tender. Luis covers it in glad wrap and suggests I get some cream from the chemist. 'Don't pick at the scab,' he says. 'Wash it with ordinary soap and warm water.' It costs me a hundred dollars.

I take my owl home on the tram. We already have a special bond.
I feel it is his nature to be supportive, nurturing. I know already that
I can tell him things; he has kind eyes. At home the cats are waiting for their dinner. I take an alprazolam and a swig of vodka and
look at the homework Winsome has set – to note down the dreams
that wake me in the middle of the night, dreams in which I am tied
up, locked up, stabbed or suffocated or thrown off a precipice while
tied up. Sometimes I'm force fed or injected or tied to a bed. There
is a lot of background jeering and laughter. I write this down, read it
through and then screw the paper up and toss it in the bin. It sounds
ridiculous.

The new psychiatrist at the Community Clinic, replacing Jim, reminds
me of an Amazon horned frog. He asks the same six questions in the
same order every week. It's obvious he's bored and he doesn't want
to be here and I don't much want to be here either, but Winsome,
as a psychologist, cannot prescribe medication or assess symptoms
medically. After the third consult he gives me a prescription for a
drug called Risperidone.

'What's this for?' I ask.

'It will settle your thinking.'

'There's nothing wrong with my thinking.'

'Okay, well, see how you feel after a few days.'

Communication between psychiatrists and patients is a complex
thing. There are many obstacles. There is a real difference between
how one should communicate with an acutely unwell patient and how
one should communicate with someone who is relatively stable. I do
not ever feel like a true 'partner' in the process of illness-management.

this paper has thick edges, like old manuscript. It has a certain seriousness. It will make a certain sound when turned ———— there has a crown of brass made to look like old gold. It speaks of having matter, of existing even when out of sight. They mutter SEN, Their extraordinariness is Black Air and it has no substance, no matter, it has no matter but it is not how nothing is — not in the way a vacuum in space is nothing.

Write: Solstice
Summer Equinox
Candles
Pendulum

Mathematics
as universal
language
Galileo

I feel instead like a recalcitrant child, rarely taken seriously and confusingly in need of discipline.

'I tried to discuss the finer points of diagnosis with him,' I say to Helen, later. 'And the potential side-effects of this new drug.' I wave the prescription high in the air. 'He responded by looking at his watch and saying he had another patient waiting to see him.'

Helen's on maternity leave from next week – for a year. I give her a bunch of multi-hued gerberas, alight, and a card that says all the meaningful things I'm too scared to say out loud. At home I look up MIMS (the list of pharmaceuticals available in Australia) for Risperidone. It is an anti-psychotic drug, indicated for the treatment of schizophrenia and related psychoses. I put the prescription in the rubbish bin.

One afternoon after work I go to the hospital to visit Anna for coffee. I have to walk past the psychiatric ward. My knees start to shake. I look through the glass door for a moment – people are shuffling, their eyes on the ground, their arms stiff by their sides. Anna's office is filled with light. She greets me with a quick hug, which I almost enjoy and I thank her for saving my life. We talk about her family and my family.

'It's a terrible thing, I guess, to watch your only child falling apart,' I say, thinking of my mother and father.

'Yes. A terrible thing. One of the worst things.'

'I don't know how to make it better for them. And they don't know how to make it better for me. We try – we spend whole days together trying so damn hard not to upset each other and not knowing what else to do or say except to wonder if the coffee's freshly ground or if it's forecast to rain.'

'Ah, but they love that you are at least *here*, to talk about the coffee and the rain,' says Anna.

My eyes flush bright for a second with tears, and then Anna's do too. She suggests the name of a psychiatrist whom I could see privately for medication and symptom review, away from the informal chaos of the Community Clinic. 'I trust him,' she says. We have coffee. When she speaks, I sit very still, and as we walk slowly back to the psychiatry wing arm in arm I feel almost human.

15

Another weekly visit with Winsome.

'What helps you stay grounded?' she asks.

'Books, music – cello – sometimes if I just play the notes with my left hand there's this feeling of the music rising up through the fingerboard.'

'You love the cello?'

'Well, I love it when Adam, my teacher, plays. Me, not so much. I've got a shitty ear for pitch. Can't hold a tune for anything as a singer. Maybe it'll get better with practice. But when Adam plays, say, Bach's Fourth Suite, the sound . . . it resonates like . . . like photons of light through water – it's the purest sort of energy. It runs right through me.'

'Is it joy?'

'I hadn't thought of it like that . . . Yeah. I think it is.'

'Can you hold onto it? Can you let go of what's happening in your mind and hold that feeling – joy – in your body?'

I consider. There's something in this room that's hard to give a simple name to. It's a kind of stillness, a kind of warm uncluttered stillness, like the room can expand and contain and hold safe anything that's said inside it. Then it occurs to me that the room being inanimate means Winsome is creating this aura, this echo of unconditional shelter.

99

I walk home. Another evening with booze and benzos and books. I'm reading *Let Us Now Praise Famous Men* by James Agee. What a fusion of art and politics, philosophy, social commentary and the wretched, desolate minutiae of human life! Of course, it's the form, the style, the juxtaposition of themes and points of view that are so unique. Some reviewer said, 'This book might just re-wire your brain.' I think I agree, all the better after a quart of whisky and some clonazepam. Rose and Henry lie on the couch beside me. The night leans in, the darkness presses.

The next day is blue and white and warm. It's a day off work. I drive to St Kilda, walk by Luna Park down to the sea, drop my bag of books on the sand and take my shoes off, let the sand run through my toes. Then I go down to the water's edge and walk into the water in my clothes, long pants and a jumper. I walk out until my feet have to leave the bottom to keep my head above the water. The water is cold with sudden patches of warmth where sunshine has penetrated. I swim slowly. My clothes flow around me like an extension of my skin; I am some kind of sea creature. I turn onto my back and drift, arms out wide. There's a nice swell this far out, but no waves. The water touches me all over like silk. If I lie so that my ears are under the water I can't hear the people in my head, just the slop and gush of the sea.

After an hour or so I come back in to shore, sit down on the sand with my clothes steaming and watch other people on the beach. There's a young man quite close to me with an enormous silver ring through the centre of his nose and a series of rings running right up and over the shells of his ears. His eyebrows are tattooed into a pattern of unfolding fern fronds. I raise my own eyebrows at him and smile.

In the evening I take the tram to a terrace house in the city. The house, including the iron lace work, is painted a deep red-brown.

Inside it's cool and dim. I join other people in the waiting room where there are old copies of the *Medical Journal of Australia* lying in a pile beside the coffee table. I read an article on 'Substance misuse in patients with acute mental illness'. The authors found that 60 per cent of patients admitted to an acute psychiatric facility in Adelaide had a co-morbid substance misuse disorder, be it with cannabis, alcohol, amphetamines, heroin or benzodiazepines. Many patients misused more than one substance. 'No shit,' I mutter out loud.

Aaron, my new psychiatrist, calls me into his consulting room. I remember him from my time in the hospital. He's rotund; short and round with a youthful face and pink cheeks and pale blonde hair. His room, on the second floor, looks like an old ballroom. It has a parquetry floor and a high ceiling. I imagine people doing the cha cha down the centre, music playing on a gramophone in the corner. Aaron asks me all the usual history-taking questions: age, marital status, parents, work, intimate relationships, family history of mental illness, personal history of mental illness, medication, alcohol and other drugs. By the end of the fifty minutes my skin is peeled back to expose my innards, my naked, painful self. I stumble outside, straight to the nearest bottle shop, keen all through the night, finally take enough lorazepam for a few hours sleep and then reel back into work the next morning.

'Japanese sushi chefs have at least fifteen different knives for the slicing of fish,' I say to Winsome. 'Did you know that?' I'm thinking about slicing my flesh. I confess to her that I've started carrying a hunting knife.

'Where did you get it?' she asks.

'Local army surplus store. It's a Dewey, for skinning, 3.5 mm thick.' I say it with pride. Winsome does not look impressed.

'Have you got it with you?'

'No, it's at home.'

'Will you bring it in and give it to me?'

I think about this. I like my knife. It lies on my bedside table at night, all cool metal, full of possibility. But Winsome is still in her chair, hands relaxed on her thighs, a string of understated pearls around her neck.

'Please go home, Kate, and bring in the knife. It's a dangerous thing to be carrying around.' She says it very clearly, quietly, so calmly, and yet her voice fills the room. 'It can never come to any good.'

I picture running the knife lightly over the tips of my fingers. Bubbles of blood, miniature red balloons form above the faint pink of my skin, slide into the circles and whorls of my fingerprint.

Then again. Could this be a good kind of leap . . . of faith . . . in someone else that she (Winsome) knows better, is wiser? Is thinking rationally? At home I wrap the Dewey knife in layers of newspaper, secure it with packing tape and drop it in an industrial rubbish bin.

On my way to work on the train I swallow several No Doze tablets, wash them down with Red Bull, follow up with several cups of strong coffee. Then in the evening I strangle the caffeine hit with benzos and alcohol and codeine. Lurching from a minor high in the morning to a semi-coma at night, I'm distilling and then diluting the people in my head. It is a simple chemistry experiment: take two of this and three of that, add half a cup of whisky, wait a while and repeat if no effect.

Zoë and I go to Brunswick Street on the weekend, wander through the shops, through the filigree jewellery, the hopelessly funky clothes.

'You'd look great in this,' I say, stroking a dark red dress.

'Nah,' she says. 'Check this out,' she holds up a sleeveless dress with a black owl sewn into the front.

'Gorgeous,' I say.

'Would you wear it?'

'Scars, dammit.'

'Dammit. Long tee underneath and opaque stockings?'

'In winter, maybe.'

'Try it on.'

'Nope. Too embarrassed. You try it on.'

She grins. 'I'm not obsessed with owls.'

We both order a double vodka and orange at the nearest pub and share our recent experiences of therapy and shrinks and medication. We listen intently to each other's stories; we laugh a lot, blackly, but shy away from tears.

I'm starting to count the days down until my next appointment with Winsome. It's Saturday, four days to go, it's Sunday, three to go. I turn up to her rooms immersed in the people in my head, insistent about the bleakness of life, stumbling over that thing called sanity. I leave with a sense of lightness, my feet firmly on the ground and a slight warmth in my heart.

'This relationship is about trust,' she says. 'Do you trust me, Kate?'

Almost, I think.

Outside Winsome's office is the sky. Oh, the sky. Falling through low bunched clouds are strands of sunlight that open out like a fan or a bird's wing stretched in flight. I walk as fast as I can to the sea – striding, breathing in . . . out . . . in . . . deep and long. Past the cafes, the windows with clothing I will never fit into, the gelato shop's tubs that look like mountain peaks in pink (berry) and pale green (pistachio) and white. Up one hill past the liberal synagogue, down another hill past the Yeshiva and the Uniting Church Hall and the op shops. There's a photo of Janet Leigh screaming on a wall with the sign 'Warning: Keep Clear' above her head.

At the edge of the sea I sit on a concrete wall. Spaced fairly equally along the railing are a group of terns, their black and white feathers drying in the sun. One of them stretches its wings and its black wing-span is thick and wide as a cape and I imagine it velvet, soft as the wind that roars up from the Southern Ocean before settling into a cushiony breeze around the bay. Sunlight is touching the water about a hundred metres from the shore and each point of light that quivers there polishes the water into cut diamonds. I can't stop smiling. Perhaps god is revealing something of heaven.

But there is a Holocaust documentary on television when I get home. It is shot in black and white. The footage is of Nazi destruction of Jewish homes and businesses, the ghettos and the camps, the horror. After it has finished I find some sticks of incense and light them. It is essential that I know something of suffering so I use the lit ends to burn a Star of David into the skin of my shoulder. It takes about an hour, it is a brand.

I visit Aaron but I can't tell him anything that matters. I look at his face and my resolve to be honest leaves me, leaves me flailing about in the minutiae of how many hours I'm sleeping, how many tablets of lithium I'm taking, while the real stuff sits beside me in a great lump on the couch. He asks questions, I'm evasive. My answers are convoluted and only slightly relevant to the topic at hand. I create pictures out of words, I rarely stop talking but nothing I say has real meaning, nothing gets at the heart of things.

'I think we're making progress,' he says at the end of fifty minutes. I pick up my bag of books and smile and walk out of his office onto Chapel Street where it is dusk, a flock of fruit bats flies low overhead quite silently. I imagine the air flowing over and under their leathery wings, keeping them afloat.

'Kate,' Winsome says. 'You've been coming here every week for six months, all through spring and summer, and you haven't once taken that enormous coat off.'

I wrap the coat tighter around me; clutch the pile of books to my chest like the characters and the writers are sitting here too.

'You must be boiling hot,' she says.

'I don't know – or at least ever notice – if I'm hot or cold.'

'That isn't normal,' she says gently.

'Isn't it?'

'Will you take Berocca?' she asks.

'What for?'

'To give your body something with nutritive value. You only have to drink it.'

I consider this. 'The body hasn't had anything of nutritive value for years.'

'Now is a good time to change that,' she looks at me directly; she holds my eyes in hers. Her eyes are not softly lit; they are darker than I've ever seen them before. They are solid, determined.

After the session I walk to the supermarket. Immediately I'm through those automatic doors the people in my head start up.

seven plus three is nine align witch you're an ugly bitch weeeeeee we're killing you killing killing killing killing

I stand just inside the doors and hit the back of my thighs with my fists to get my legs to move forwards. It's hard not to look at the ground – if I look up, into the faces of other people, then they can see me, if I look at the ground, I'm invisible. I walk through the fruit and vegetables, ominous in their gleaming piles. I know there are cameras in here, behind the little bulbs of dark blue glass. Monitoring.

Berocca is in the medicinal section near the back of the store. I keep my head down and promptly collide with some children, one of whom sits on the polished linoleum and begins to cry.

'God, sorry,' I say. 'Sorry.' My vision goes all blurry, I can just see a parent in the distance and I turn and walk out fast, before the monitoring people can arrest me.

16

It's autumn. The plane trees outside my window at work are losing their leaves. The air has an edge to it, a raciness, the dark descends quickly. The exotic dark. It's mania weather. I talk and walk fast, I write fast. I'm reading five books at once; I sing in my head while carrying on a conversation, I compliment people.

'You're looking sexy today,' I say to my manager. He stops and half-smiles. After work I walk all the way home. There is magic and colour in the air and I may burst from my skin; inhabit something larger in both space and time. Nights like these, the boundaries of everything shift around me. Walls, floors, sound – especially sound. Music saturates the room, clings to my skin, flows like fine wine. I am a risk-taker, a Russian-roulette-player. As soon leap off a mountain as walk down the street. I am cool – I like Nine Inch Nails really loud, and the Tea Party, Jane's Addiction, Rancid, punk-anything, acid and flame. Each note is a colour, there is colour everywhere, tonight I am DIVINE.

Arthur Boyd created a series of paintings about Nebuchadnezzar, King of Babylon, exiler, despot. In one, he is painted from above, all deepest yellow, his arms outstretched and his fingers grasping the gold air. He is dying. I fall in love with it and ring the South Australian Art Gallery: can they make me a reproduction? I need it. It is essential. All meaning is to be found in this painting.

I try to explain it to Winsome, sitting on the very edge of the chair, my lap piled with books, earphones around my neck still playing.

'Everything is very beautiful,' I say. 'Look at the way light is stuttering through your glass ornament – it's all about the blue and then it's white and then it's gone! I can't keep up with the pace of light, I think it's extraordinary that we can see light at all; I wish I'd studied special relativity but my brain simply refuses to hold onto the facts. There's definitely something wrong with some of my neurones, though I'd secretly prefer to visit an art gallery because art is where light gets to show herself off, don't you think? And so I wonder—'

'Kate,' says Winsome. 'You're keeping me entertained, but I don't think you are well. Have you got an appointment with Aaron?'

I sigh and stand and pace along the wall by the window. 'Tomorrow.'

'Good. What are you doing tonight?'

'Painting my fence blue. Blue is such a universal colour. It's honest, but its depths are full of mystery. Isn't it amazing that it can be both at the same time?'

'Yes. How did you get here?'

'Tram, which is excellent—'

'Kate,' says Winsome again. I stop pacing. 'Come and sit down.'

'I can't, I really can't, look!' I stand on my tiptoes and throw my arms out wide; I'm silhouetted like a star against the window for all the people in the street to see.

The next day I put on a lot of make up and go to work an hour early. I drink ten cups of coffee. I do jumping jacks in the toilet with my headphones on. I wonder if the BDSM house will take me on as a Mistress.

In the evening I visit Aaron. 'How are you?' he asks, as usual. I stand in front of him with my hands on my hips, sticking my pelvis out.

'Do you kiss with tongue?' I say, and then I start giggling and I can't stop, I keep giggling and now tears are seeping out from the sides of my eyes and smudging the mascara I put on this morning for the first time in years. I'm rocking back and forth on my feet, laughing and crying in equal measure. Aaron doesn't say anything; he reaches over to the phone on his desk and rings the CAT team.

'Are you taking your lithium?' he asks, mid-conversation.

'Of course,' I say. I have no idea where the bottle of lithium is – somewhere in my bedroom, probably under the bed where the cats sometimes pee.

He hangs up the phone. 'Are you sleeping?'

'Thorough waste of time.' I sit down. 'I do miss dreaming though. You know Freud thought that dream-life was just as important as waking-life for the illumination of the psyche. I think I agree with him, well I do at this particular moment, God, your taste in art is awful, Aaron.'

'Kate,' says Aaron. 'I would like you to take one of these – now.' He pulls a blister pack of tablets out of his top desk drawer. His desk is old, made of some wood with lines and whorls and stained dark chestnut.

'What's this?' I ask.

'Seroquel. It's an atypical anti-psychotic. Also good for hypomania.' He stands and says, 'Just stay there a minute.' I sway from side to side on the chair singing the Cat Power song 'Good Woman.' Aaron gives me a glass of water and a round, white tablet.

'How much?' I ask.

'200 milligrams,' he says.

I stare at it. The tablet is changing shape in my palm. It's circular, then oval, then it expels a part of itself and becomes two tablets.

I stare at Aaron. 'What are you doing?'

'I'm trying to stabilise your mood.'

He waits, leaning on his desk with his arms crossed. The creases in his shirt catch the light and shine. I smile.

'Take the Seroquel, please.'

The tablet is furry round the edges where it has mixed with my sweat. I put it in my mouth and take a swig of water and swallow down its bitterness.

'Happy?'

'Thank you,' he says. 'The CAT team are going to visit you later tonight.'

'Excellent,' I say and stand up and bow so that my forearms touch the ground. 'It has been a pleasure doing business with you, Sir.'

Aaron almost smiles.

The CAT team this evening consists of Angela and Gary. Angela is eight months pregnant.

'Can I use your loo?' she asks as soon as I open the door. I sit on the floor with a pile of books in my lap, mainly poetry, and keep reading while the CAT team ask questions.

'Can we have your car keys, Kate?' asks Angela. 'We're worried about you driving too fast. What do you think?'

'Yeah, yeah. Probably.'

I can hear someone singing, '. . . Beware! Beware! His flashing eyes! His floating hair!'

'Who is singing?' I ask looking around the room and into the corners of the ceiling.

'We'd like you to take a week off work.'

'Ah hah.'

'Here's some seroquel for you to take with your lithium in the morning.' The tablets, in their silver casing, look like tiny UFOs. I put them in my pocket and follow Angela and Gary down the stairs and out into the street where night holds fast to the sky.

'Check out the stars!' I say, whirling around.

'Go to bed, Kate. We'll see you tomorrow.' I wait until their car turns into High Street, and then I drop the seroquel in one of the big green rubbish bins out the front of my block of flats. I don't sleep.

Seroquel (quetiapine) is one of a class of drugs known as atypical antipsychotics. It binds to serotonin receptors and dopamine receptors in the brain and is effective for people with schizophrenia and bipolar disorder, particularly those with acute mania. Seroquel is sedating. It slows thought, reins in excessive activity and improves sleep, but I have no intention of taking anything that might curb this flight.

In the morning I go into work as usual. Rather than reading articles on childhood asthma from the *Journal of Paediatrics and Child Health*, I spend the day writing poetry. I'm seized with the desirability of words: their ability to sculpt new worlds, fantastical and pure.

The CAT team visit in the early evening and give me some more seroquel, which I deposit in the rubbish bin on my way into the city. I've got a bottle half full of Coke and half full of vodka. Behind Safeway there is a small park with some children's play equipment and a fluorescent light on the wall that flickers. Sitting in a circle on the grass are two old men in jeans and two young men in tracksuits.

'Hiya,' I say, finding a spot on the grass.

'Hey,' says one of the young men. The old ones nod their heads in my direction. They've got a couple of joints going between them.

'Got any money, love?'

'Heaps.'

'Get us some smokes?'

'Sure!' I'm in Safeway and I stride fast up and down the aisles with their glorious colours and I buy five kinds of nail polish and two cartons of Marlboro Reds and then I go next door for a slab of VB. Back outside the wind has picked up.

The men aren't keen to share their marijuana, but they take the booze and the smokes as I go around shaking everyone by the hand.

'Would you like some nail polish?' I ask one of the old men. He has a hatched beard; he's wearing an army coat fraying in long lines of cotton at the wrists. I offer the little bottles, Electric Pink and Royal Rajah Ruby and Lacy Not Racy. He laughs and shakes his head at me and lights a cigarette.

I spin off into a club down the street, with its door open, music and light spilling out. The music is hip-hop, loud, with a good bass. I stand next to a couple who look Latino – they've got such shiny eyes and hair, and such silky skin I could run my hands like honey all over them. I dance with the nearly empty bottle of vodka and Coke in one hand. At 2 a.m. they turn the music off, though I'm still dancing (the only one still dancing), wet inside my coat, blisters running up my heels.

'God, that was good,' I say, as one of the staff ushers me out. I stand on the pavement, stick my hand out for a passing taxi.

'Do you know any other languages?' I ask the driver, whose name is Alekso.

'Macedonian,' he says.

'Say "I love you" in Macedonian.'

He pauses, looks across at me in the gloom of the taxi with his brown eyes that are catching the dobs of streetlights and reflecting them. 'Te sakam,' he says.

'Te sakam, Alekso,' I say.

17

At home I write PROMETHEUS in red in one of my notebooks. I gather a pile of paper, bills and letters; some unopened, and kindle it in my courtyard with a match. The flame skirts the edges of the paper like it's teasing, then it flares as it finds oxygen in the night air. I crouch in close; I can feel heat on my eyes, stands of hair singe round my forehead with a tiny phzz. This is holy fire, the sort that Moses encountered on Mt Horeb. There are faces in the flame, jokers and fire angels, Prometheus himself with his half-eaten liver and Munch's scream. I don't blink for so long the fine layer of liquid over my eyes evaporates, leaving them dry as hard-boiled eggs. I try to kiss the flame, touch it, hold it, but it's slippery, it lights upon a spot in the night, sucks the air, is gone.

Instead of sleeping, I sit in bed, reading. There's a sort of buzzing in my head like tinnitus, but more tactile; inside the beehive in my skull the bees are edgy. I get up and look at my face in the mirror. My eyes are all pupils, black and cavernous. The whites are shot red.

Someone is singing, 'Beware! Beware! His flashing eyes! His floating hair!'

On the train to work people are staring at the way I manage to curl air in through my nostrils and blow it out again through my mouth, coloured and alive. I'm creating life from a conglomeration of gases: nitrogen, oxygen, argon, carbon dioxide. Is this what God did when he created the firmament of the heavens and the celestial spheres? Is this what it is to be holy?

At work I write about orchids.

We smouldered; crysalised in the humid earth, mothy, pure. We suckled on sun. Air entered us like semen. Do not think of us as flowers; we pollinate more than stamen and xylem. We luminesce, we distil chlorophyll, we dream in vanilla and lime. We are pubescent and pendulous; nigrescent. We radiate. In the night entwined among ourselves, old sunlight congeals in our veins. Do they excite you, our swollen heads? Today you will salivate over our fibrillose lips, our scalloped throats, and we will finger you, infect the colour around you. Perhaps we have teeth. All of us – bromelades, cattleya, oncidiae – invented the meaning of life before your species was even conceived, dissolved it deep in our nuclei, let it swell there while we copulated with glutinous pollen and bees and lust.

air prayer beware

Of the four classical elements in alchemy, air is symbolic of action and purity, it is hot and wet. It follows that all I need to stay alive is air. I hold this revelation, this epiphany, folded to my breast as I would a love letter. Instead of having lunch I buy a leather desk chair for around three months' salary.

In the evening, Gary and Angela visit and I take the opportunity to wonder about the difference between theology and divinity and the meaning of divine, and whether divinity of the spirit is inevitably corrupted by the mind, but all Gary and Angela are interested in is seroquel.

'You don't appear to be slowing down,' Angela says, sitting on the very edge of the lounge chair with knees wide apart to accommodate her belly.

'I know, it's fabulous, isn't it? Maybe I'm immune. Seriously, what if I've got special liver enzymes that metabolise Seroquel in the blink of an eye?' I wink at her and smile.

'I don't think so,' she says, looking at Gary.

'Okay,' says Gary. 'Here's your evening dose. We're going to watch you take it. Go and get some water.'

On the way to the kitchen the people in my head and I agree that seroquel is not a good idea. This space, this time, this realm is an ideal grace. It is pure, as vital as blood, and boundless. I return with a glass of water and Gary slips two white tablets from their silver casing into my palm. I tip my head back and flick the tablets over my back teeth to the inside of my right cheek. I drink the water, letting it slide down the left side of my mouth and throat. I smile at both of them and take the glass back to the kitchen and remove the soggy, bitter-white mush, my head inclined a fragile inch. Mavis, my big black cat, opens her eyes wide, wide.

The remainder of the night passes. I wake up on the floor in the living room with bits of fluff in my mouth and my head on a copy of *The Diary of Frida Kahlo*. Frida painted in oils mostly, so I stop off on the way to work at Eckersley's Art and buy tubes of Cadmium Red, Vermillion, a bottle of sun-refined linseed oil, two flat hog-hair-bristle brushes and several stretched canvases. By evening, however, it is clear that my real vocation lies with the women of the night in Greeves Street, St Kilda – there is something in the dark sea air, something amorous and slightly racy.

inject connect sex

'Where or what is your brightest part?' I ask the woman sitting opposite me on the tram. 'Would you say it was your soul?'

A young man stands on the pavement in front of the National Theatre. He's very thin, very feminine (and beautiful). I sit down with my back to the dusky-pink bricks and stare at the veins in his forearms, lines of pillowed-blood, perfect under the skin.

'I could fall into your eyes and die,' I say.

He looks at me and frowns. 'You right?'

'I said, I could fall into your eyes and die.'

'Look, I don't even know you, just piss off out of my space.'

'Jesus! What if we're buried together? What're you going to do then?'

He walks away down Carlisle Street in his tall black-heeled boots and I reel in the other direction up Barkly Street and then left into Grey Street. The Sacred Heart Mission is shut for the night; the iron gates are closed and quiet. On the roof of one of the buildings are three thick cream crosses; on the other building there are five. Three crosses for the holy trinity and the three states of matter. Five crosses for the four limbs of the body and the head in the centre. The upper windows of the op shop and the main building have eyes with stained glass irises.

all the colours burst amid echoes raaaaw

'Roar!' I yell at the night.

At home I open all the curtains in my flat and light all the candles and put them on windowsills. I light fists of sandalwood incense and arrange them in vases on either side of my newly created shrine to Dylan Thomas. The television is on and the radio is on and the CD player in my room is on because I can absorb sound in all three dimensions and process each independently. There are books covering the floor, lining the walls, strung across the ceiling.

'You haven't been taking your seroquel or your lithium, have you?' asks Angela, when she and Gary arrive ten minutes later.

'No, but I'm not trying to be difficult, I'm really not, it's because I'm at one with all the world: the physical, the mortal, the metaphysical. Think of natural fractals: no matter at which level you look – macro or micro or nano – they're perfect, and I understand – it's like when the solo treble hits high C – it's rapture.'

Gary and Angela confer.

'We're going to take you for a review at the hospital,' Gary says.

'Why?'

'We don't want you doing anything silly, anything you might regret.'

'This is the craziness of the world: there's never a good answer to the question why.'

Angela goes around blowing out candles while Gary rings ahead on his mobile and then he takes my keys and locks the flat and Angela walks me down the stairs to their sensible, white car and we drive very sensibly (very slowly) to the hospital.

In the seventeenth and eighteenth centuries, mania was variously described as a frenzy without fever, an insensibility tense with internal vibrations, a secret fire of open and burning flame, an agitation of cerebral fluid. Early physicians theorised that the cause of the illness lay in the 'continuous and violent movement of heat, the spirits and the humours.'

At the hospital I introduce myself to the night staff and ask one of the nurses whose eyes are bewitching me if I can give her a hug, which she allows, arms straight down by her sides. I'm given a measuring cup of dark red syrup and four white tablets.

'The blood of Christ, the body of Christ, Amen,' I say.

Because I am thus far compliant, I'm given a room on the main ward opposite the staff station. It's very white – walls, bed, linen, floor – but I have Dylan Thomas with me for illumination, all of his honey-coloured words.

In the morning I stride round and round the courtyard listening to the Stone Roses on repeat until I'm called in to see Aaron, who works on the public ward in the mornings and sees his private patients in the afternoons.

'The CAT team have filled me in,' he says.

'Beware! Beware! His flashing eyes! His floating hair!'

I turn around to see who's singing.

'Who's singing?' I ask.

'We'll have to give you an injection in the buttocks if you don't settle down soon,' Aaron says.

Zoë comes to visit – it's fantastic to see her and I go round introducing her to everyone.

'How are you?' she asks.

'Who so regardeth dreams is like him that catcheth at a shadow and followeth after the wind. That's from Ecclesiastes,' I reply.

'Right,' she says. 'Your cords are on backwards.'

We're out in the courtyard, smoking. 'Hah!' I pull my jeans down and my shirt up and stand for a moment in my underwear, feeling the air move on my breasts and legs.

'The tax office phoned yesterday,' I say. 'They're developing a kind of new philosophy; it's to do with how they assess whether people have to pay tax or not, I mean, there's got to be more to it than just how much you earn, right? Circus performers shouldn't have to pay tax and I'm going to write the new policy.'

'Okay,' says Zoë.

I start pacing, 'That white cat is invading me.'

'There's no cat, Kate.'

'No? But there are different degrees of light; it's all about angles and diffraction, so there could be a cat; you just can't see it.'

Staff walk me inside to Aaron's consulting room.

'How are you today?' he asks.

'I have absolutely no idea,' I say. 'I'm wrinkled with drugs, unplug the firebug or we'll all go up in flames.'

'How did you sleep last night?'

'Queen Mab raped me. Hah! The fairies' midwife!'

'Are your thoughts still racing?'

'I don't know what they're doing, ô sales fous ô sales fous ô sales fous ô sales fous—'

Aaron interrupts me, 'What are you saying?'

'O filthy lunatics . . . Rimbaud. Yes? No.'

I spend hours in the art room writing columns of words that rise from the page into strange spirit phrases and engulf me.

At least twice a day I burst (literally) into tears like I've had a frontal lobotomy, and at least twice a day, for no particular reason, rage rises up through my innards and strangles me about the throat so that I take to stuffing a pillow in my mouth.

This morning words are not to be trusted, their power is omnipresent, they bruise me. I can't sit still long enough to hover over more than a phrase. Aaron responds by increasing the seroquel.

At lunch a very tall young woman is standing right in the middle of my personal space.

'I know you from somewhere,' she says, staring.

'Really? Are you a reincarnation?'

Spangle

a sequined ether, a processional
stanza of irises! of Eyes that
part off the eyes that irradiate
immortality and hysteria in a
single flutter. A BUTTERED FLOWER —
All the flare in the udder, the
centre, the stanza. As good as a
solstice (the tilt of the earth's
axis is — — — —) effectively a
flower dipped in butter, wet.
Soaking and pure 's yellow-
ness new Messiah. The way Grace
is pure, never fragmentary, sure &
always sure of Immortality.
Purer than white, pure as urine
and pasturised milk (I can't smell him)
I could take all this now and stuff
it in my mouth and chew it
into a myth and then let it
ooze into my brain
            (defying gravity)
the way lemon juice flows up into
tears and tears flare in the
sun and make a prism and
all the colours — an eye, a stars
(Did God know this?) Belong in the sky.

'You're a spy.'

'Nope, not today.'

'You're a spy!' she shouts, and suddenly she kicks me, hard, right on the tender-bone of my shin. I never find out her name. By the time my heart slows down, she is marched off by two staff to the High Dependency Unit.

Aaron finds me later, pacing around the courtyard in bare feet.

'How are you?' he asks.

if the clock strikes nine times shout the people in my head.

'If the clock strikes nine times,' I say.

the head of a swallow shall lie at your feet

'The head of a swallow shall lie at your feet.'

and your toes will burn slowly

'And your toes will burn slowly,'

will smoulder black and red

'Will smoulder black and red,'

the stench of your skin shall never leave you

'The stench of your skin shall never leave you.'

'Mmm,' Aaron says.

'You can shoot me if you like,' I say. 'It won't matter.' And then I sit for a moment next to Steve, who has an extraordinary halo of orange hair reaching in spirals into the middle distance. He doesn't speak to other patients. I watch him put a cigarette between his lips and light it. As he inhales, saliva on his lower lip gets caught by the sun and catches fire.

'Shining and burning,' I whisper to him, but he doesn't acknowledge me.

A nurse arrives with my midday syrup.

'Barukh atah adonai eloheinu melekh ha'olam, she hakol nih'yeh bid'varo,' I say, and swallow.

'Are you Jewish?' asks the nurse.

'No, but when I was twenty-four I wanted to (a) play Méditation by Jules Massenet on the cello, and (b) understand fire. So you see?'

'Not really,' she says, frowning.

'Nerves are blue, nerves are yellow,' I say.

if you watch your heartbeat you may survive

Someone is singing.

'I'm so confused.' I start twisting my head round with my hands; if I twist hard enough, I may be able to wrench it off my neck. Anna finds me thus, sits down beside me and quietly takes both my hands in hers.

'My eyes are full of glass,' I tell her. We sit in silence until Steve starts talking out loud to his voices, who appear to be plaguing him. He paces along the end of the courtyard over the spreading shrubs, hands in fists.

'No!' he shouts. 'No!' The veins in his neck fill and pulse. Sonia, a dual-diagnosis patient (intellectual disability and mental illness), walks past in a short floral skirt; her naked lower buttocks hang down like paired cauliflower heads.

18

My boss rings. He is fairly irritated that I disappeared from work without notice. I attempt an explanation, but the people in my head are interfering with my hearing – I pick up every third word he says, in between they shrill –

asphyxiate decapitate dilate weeeeeeee

Consequently he doesn't make any sense.

'You don't have any leave left,' he says.

'I think I'll resign,' I say. 'Yeah, I want to resign. I'm not wasting any more time with work.'

'That might be best,' he says.

The birds are singing; such a vivid sound. I've become a surge of red, a soul stretched tight, caught and bound by the shadows in the trees, the trees whose green feeds me over and over, whose light crazes skin into a thousand tributaries, like the visions of one, or millions. I walk into the common room where a woman I haven't seen before is standing quite alone. I lean against a wall and watch her. She holds herself together with her arms and hands that reach tight under her breasts and keep her from fragmenting. The flatness of her eyes stretches on and on and her breath is lifeless air, and her soul, risen to heaven and spurned, has fallen back into her body and burned.

'Ashes. Dust,' I say softly and open my mouth wide and eat into my gathered palms.

Two more weeks pass in which everything – person, sky, air, dream, eye – is the most significant entity, the most vital piece of existence on earth. My parents visit, Zoë visits, Tanya and Chris visit. It's wonderful to see them.

'What have you been doing?' they ask.

'I've no idea,' I answer. 'Have I been here long?' My voice is dry and hoarse.

'I've got laryngitis,' I tell Aaron.

'No,' he says, 'You've merely worn your voice out.' I give him a squashed version of the finger.

Winsome rings, calm and velvety, and I explain about the white cat and the tax office, the slow burning of toes and how yesterday the saliva on Steve's lip caught fire which is remarkable, given that saliva isn't usually flammable.

'What's happening about your job?' Winsome asks.

'The job? No idea.'

Margaret, the ward social worker, helps me apply for unemployment benefits. The Department of Family and Community Services calls unemployment benefits, labour–market-assistance-related-income-support, which makes me laugh. My handwriting appears on the page wobbly as a snail trail; my eyes flutter among words but refuse to focus.

There is such a shortage of acute psychiatric beds that patients are almost always discharged mildly unwell. Readmission after another crisis in the community is not uncommon.

As my father walks with me across the road to his car, I lunge towards the traffic, heady with the possibility of flight or at least of invincibility in the face of collision. My father circumnavigates my right upper arm with both hands and holds on like a python till we're on the other side.

The floor of my little flat appears to be alive. Piles of books, piles of photographs and magazines look like squat bodies, their heads made of CDs stacked without their cases. There are Chinese incense sticks, pages of writing, notebooks, three atlases – all open, drawings and paintbrushes and cigarettes and empty vodka bottles and spilt red wine. A body made of five astronomy textbooks is next to one of four dictionaries and a King James Bible. The largest of the piles is unopened mail. There are clumps of black words cut out from newspapers and words stuck all over the walls, crookedly. Beneath them is a poster of the Hebrew aleph-bet. There are puddles of candle wax in murky green and pink on the window ledges and splotches of candle wax on the carpet that look like burst fireworks. A silver menorah I have never seen before is balanced on ee cummings' *73 Poems* and a copy of the Qur'an. Everything is covered in a fine rain of ash.

My parents clean quietly and graciously. The pages of some books are stuck together with nail polish and are thrown out, but the nail polish on the covers of others has advanced in the way of Joan Miró, and must therefore be classed as art. The phone is off and the gas and electricity are off and my father arranges for re-connection and pays the mound of bills.

It takes another five weeks to find my right mind. Initially the CAT team visit every evening to monitor medication and mood. Time re-asserts itself into seconds and minutes and hours, trees are no longer animate in the way of animals, my speech resumes a normal rate and flow. Most importantly, the manic chaos of thought is filtered by my frontal lobe – flight of ideas and inappropriateness is recognised somewhere in my brain as flight of ideas and inappropriateness. The shine over everything is muted into simple sunlight or shade and the colour of a post box ceases to set my heart racing.

I take the tram to Port Melbourne and walk east along the beach. In places the tide is right up to the stonewall and I splash through early winter water and my shoes leave a momentary impression in the sand. Ah, impermanence. Seagulls call out. The wind is vigorous, there's sand now in my mouth and hair and sand stuck to the wet ends of my jeans. I keep my mouth shut and breathe and smile at the rawness of it – sea and sky. The light is changing from sharp white to a pensive ivory and though the sea and wind are endlessly shifting, there's a certain kind of stillness in the repeat of the waves.

Winsome and I reflect.

'It's good to see you out of hospital,' she says. 'How are you?'

'Unemployed. But also un-mad.'

'Hmm.' She looks at me for a while, not staring, just looking. Her eyes are clear; their touch doesn't hurt my eyes, or my skin, or my heart.

'I fucked up,' I say.

Winsome shifts slightly in her chair.

'I . . . um . . .'

'Were you taking your lithium?' she asks.

I sway back and forth on the couch.

'As prescribed? Every day?'

'No.'

We sit. And my stupidity oozes down between my legs like menstrual blood and onto the wooden floor. It is the darkest, darkest red.

'And now?'

'Consequences,' I say. 'No money, no sense of usefulness, no sense of mattering.'

'You matter to your family. You matter to your friends.'

I nod. 'And they're so precious and I love them, but . . . it's like I'm drifting miles out to sea.'

Her eyes say she understands.

'And I can't trust my brain, which is really frigging awful.'

'Yes.'

'It's awful.' I pull at my hair.

'Well it seems to me essential that you take your lithium as prescribed, every day.' She pauses. 'In a sense having a mental illness is no different from having diabetes. You take your medication in the same way diabetics take their insulin, and you keep on taking it until your physical body gives out and you die of something else.'

Somewhere, in the uncharted depths of grey and white matter, a part of my brain is blindingly aware that she is right.

19

Unemployment. One day falls into another, all a kind of bare grey. The cloudy sky slides together with the horizon. Bliss is a cup of barista-ed coffee. Bliss is a rainbow lorikeet flying up from the grass right in front me, so close his fiery chest heats my face and I can hear the flrrrr of his wings.

My biological clock keeps odd time. I wake at midday to feed the cats, get out of bed properly at three in the afternoon and at two AM I'm at the 24-hour supermarket for coffee beans. For the remainder of the night I drink coffee and crunch up chocolate-coated coffee beans like a horse and read and sometimes I write odd, jerky poems that are really a series of questions though they don't quite make sense as either questions or poems.

Friends from my former workplace in cancer research shout me lunch every few weeks and we chat about art and friends and football and family . . . all the normal conversational sorts of things. With them I feel less superfluous, more human. Jane, the director of the department, suggests I try a yoga class.

'Exercise? Are you completely mad?'

'It's not just exercise,' she says. 'It's about the body connecting with the mind and the mind connecting with the soul.'

I roll my eyes. 'Exercise.'

128

Walking home, I pass the local Iyengar yoga studio. There's a sheaf of pamphlets in a plastic box out the front and I take one, stick it in my bag and forget about it. A day later there's a postcard amongst the mail – a photograph of two old, wrinkly hands pressed together, palms touching, fingers pointing up. Underneath it says Namaste. I bow and say 'Namaste' back to the hands and go inside and uncork a bottle of merlot and pull out the yoga pamphlet.

The studio has a certain feel – a warmth that is more than the sum of the temperature, the wooden floor and sunlight through the high windows. People are lying or sitting cross-legged on mats along the walls. Some have cotton belts around their legs, some have blankets and bolsters. It is quiet.

'The purpose of all yoga is, according to the 2000-year-old text by Patanjali, to restrain the fluctuations of the mind and bring greater self knowledge,' says Thomas, our teacher for the twelve-week beginner program. 'You'll learn to respect your body and be alive in your body. It will become a vehicle for self-exploration.'

'You need the CAT team, love,' I whisper. I'm sitting in the corner of the room and one of the double-braided ropes bolted to the wall is pressing hard into my back.

'Stand erect with your feet together,' says Thomas. 'Stretch your toes like a fan on the floor. Make sure your weight is even on both feet.'

I've never considered my feet.

'Tuck in your waist. Create as much space as you can between your pelvis and rib-cage.'

Waist. Pelvis. Space.

'Open up the chest.'

I breathe in.

Feel the opening of the chest.'

Heart, lungs, breath, beat.

'Stretch the spine from lower back to neck. Keep your head centred over your legs.'

Vertebrae, disks, nerves.

'Bring your attention to the alignment of your body,' Thomas says. Then he says nothing for about a minute, and I'm left with a dawning, surprising, conscious kind of proprioception.

Class ends in corpse pose, which in theory is a time for relaxation and quiet reflection. The people in my head mutter and I can't close my eyes in case they catch me unawares, but as I lie here on my back, covered in thick, heavy blankets . . .

slow . . .

slowly . . . my limbs loosen and fall away.

I'm warm, connected to the floor and at the same time, floating. B.K.S Iyengar says, 'the student's body assumes numerous forms of life found in creation – from the lowliest insect to the most perfect sage.'

'Who are the important men in your life?' asks Winsome.

'My father.'

'Anyone else?'

'Marc Chagall and Leonardo da Vinci.'

'Who else?'

'Bach and Schubert, Arvo Pärt, Andre Kertész, oh – and Faulkner of course, Patrick White . . .'

'They're all dead, Kate.'

'No no – Arvo Pärt's alive, he lives in Estonia and he's the greatest modern composer. Have you ever heard his piece, Tabula Rasa? Sublime.'

'I think you know that's not the point.'

'Yeah.' I bow my head, close my eyes. Then the shaking. 'Shit. Weird?'

'No. You're scared?'

'Yes.' The shaking.

'Of intimacy?'

Yes.

'You're safe here. You are safe,' says Winsome. She pauses. 'Intimacy is about being your real self in the presence of someone else.'

I nod.

'For you, I think, we are working towards uncovering some really nurturing parts of your self that will enable you to feel more at home in your own skin. That will do for the moment.'

When I leave her office I breathe all the way in, I breathe. Opening my chest, feeling the anterior ribs, pectoral muscles, cold air like manna.

At home my friend Tanya hands me a banana. I look at its skin, suspiciously. I sniff it; hold it by its blackening tip. Then I snap off the end and peel it. The banana must have the ability to release molecules into the air like perfume because ripe banana smell is everywhere. I touch its pale flesh and one of the fibrous strings comes loose. I pull all of them one by one so they hang down around it like a waterfall.

'Eat the bloody thing,' says Tanya, laughing. I bite and hold and chew. It has a surprisingly fresh taste – somewhat untainted – rain and earth and sunshine. I smile. It's the first piece of fruit I've eaten in three years.

In class we practise warrior pose and tree pose and I learn something about strength and something about stillness and the potential of the two together. It feels good.

'With reflectiveness and self awareness,' says Thomas, quietly, 'your yoga practice becomes a mirror to the self. Your body is an instrument with which to express your mental and spiritual being.'

The people in my head laugh and laugh—

yeah you bitch you're a fucking nutcase ha ha ha break your fingers go on do it we said do it

'Bring your consciousness to your core. Feel the lift running up the back leg, across the belly and chest and into the arms.'

The class is quiet and concentrated, all of us gazing forward.

Every time I leave standing straighter, walking taller. It feels good.

I get to the supermarket in the late morning, along with mothers and prams and old women with walking frames – beginnings and endings – and I find the fruit and vegetable aisle and buy carrots, tangelos, pink lady apples. Back home I discover the kinaesthetic pleasure of fruit and vegetables – their extraordinary evolution of colour and shape and texture and taste, and I begin crunching up raw carrots like a horse, instead of coffee beans and chocolate.

Aaron monitors the high-dose lithium with regular blood tests. The side effects sit somewhere between nuisance and aggravation: nausea, thirst, pissing a lot (a consequence of the thirst), lethargy, hand tremor. And my mind is slow. I have no spark. Even my attempts at humour are dreary.

'This drug is fucked up,' I say to Winsome.

'Pardon?'

'Sorry. I mean I'm not sure if the benefits outweigh the adverse effects.'

'Kate, it's certainly not perfect and I'm sorry you have to go through this, really I am, but we have some insight into the pattern of your illness, don't you think?'

'Yes.'

'So please trust me when I say you must take your lithium. Otherwise you will become unwell again. And I sense that there is a sliver of trust . . .?'

I smile suddenly and the room floods. 'Yes.'

A couple of candles are sometimes lit in the otherwise dim foyer of the yoga studio. I love their cylindrical light.

Andy is our new Wednesday teacher. His body is all muscle. His posture is that of a ballet dancer and he moves like perfectly co-ordinated fluid. I can't help grinning, watching him.

20

Money is a real problem. Some of us with long-term mental illness are lucky enough to be financially supported or assisted by family and friends. My parents are paying the mortgage and most of my bills and I don't know how I'd manage without them. The fortnightly government allowance is swallowed up by food and groceries and cat food and the occasional book. I haven't walked into a clothing shop or a shoe shop or a department store for months. Hiring a DVD once a week is cheaper than the cinema.

To save money I pare my diet down to raw carrots, mandarins, spinach leaves and steamed rice with chilli. I drink black coffee instead of whisky. I lose a lot of weight. My blood glucose and cholesterol normalise after the years of subsisting on chocolate. Sometimes I faint if I stand up too quickly.

When one of my former colleagues in cancer research goes on long service leave, I'm offered a job as her replacement for three months. I feel somewhat re-born just at the thought of being involved in something that matters, in having a sense of purpose, in contributing. I'm also nervous; scared of performing poorly or making mistakes or of it somehow being obvious to others that I've once or twice gone mad.

I suspect that most of my workmates know I've been in a psychiatric institution, because that kind of gossip travels and I've never asked those who know me well to keep it secret. It is painful that I can't discuss what happened (whatever it was) frankly, like I would a hip replacement or even a hysterectomy. It is painful and somewhat awkward – this thing left unsaid yet present.

But I settle in uneventfully and I work hard and the best parts of the day become the times a group of us hang out together and relax – morning coffee, lunch, drinks on a Friday night at a bar up the road.

'Whatcha doing on the weekend?' we ask each other after the third beer.

'Alpine hiking,' says Deborah.

We groan in admiration.

'Sleeping,' says Jess.

'Strip club,' says Adrian.

'Adrian's horny,' we say, slapping his shoulders and knees. As the only man in a sea of women, he loves teasing us, and we him.

'Let's all go!' I say.

Adrian laughs . . . blushes.

'Gross,' say Jess.

'Why?' I say.

She frowns, mocking shock. 'Watch it.'

Later in the evening I settle into a state of nice, warm, alcohol-fuelled disinhibition. We're mulling over religion and science. 'Purring, for example,' I say randomly. 'What evolutionary benefit does purring have?'

'What?' says Jess.

'Seriously.'

'Dunno. You're weird.'

'Am so not. Am. Yeah.'

Jess gets up for another round of drinks. 'Hey,' she says, turning back to me. 'Love ya.'

'Love ya,' I say, thrilled. Quietly.

My work portfolio covers clinical trials of new and hopefully better therapeutics in leukaemia, lung cancer, breast cancer and prostate cancer. Some of the novel agents are drugs, others involve a new radiotherapy technique or a new surgical technique or a combination. We educate patients and families, provide support and collect clinical data. Obviously, the ability of a new therapy to treat or cure cancer is paramount, but we spend a lot of time assessing adverse events as well as efficacies. That is, talking with, and examining patients to see if the new treatments are affecting them adversely, and if so, what action we can take.

One of my patients is a young woman with breast cancer concerned about her fertility after chemotherapy. There's a mother of three young children who can't get out of bed in the morning because her haemoglobin is so low and a twenty-one-year old who has devastatingly relapsed after a bone marrow transplant. Some days at work are uplifting and others bring great sadness.

Richard was on his second honeymoon when he noticed blood in the toilet. He didn't tell his new wife, didn't want to worry her. Didn't tell her that he had booked in for a colonoscopy when they got home. Didn't know how to tell her when the biopsy result came back as cancer. Richard's wife hates hospitals – both her parents died in a hospital – so Richard attends his weekly appointments for chemotherapy alone.

Richard is forty-nine. He has a full time job, a new wife and two teenage sons. He has bowel cancer that has spread to his liver and lungs.

Every Wednesday at nine in the morning, Richard is sitting up straight in his chemotherapy chair with the newspaper and a cup of tea.

'Morning Kate,' he says brightly.

'Morning Richard. How are you?'

'Excellent.'

'Yeah?' I sit down beside his chemo chair.

'Yeah.' His face is more grey than pale. Exhausted.

I learn forward just a little.

'Well . . . you know how it is . . .' he says.

'How are the nights?'

He folds up his newspaper and looks at me. After a while, he says, 'Long.'

'How much sleep are you getting?'

'Not much.'

'Pain?'

'Yep.'

'Where?'

'Back, tummy, lower down.'

'Worse that last week?'

'Yeah.'

'What else?'

'Oh, the usual. Nausea.'

'Anything else?'

'Just can't get off to sleep.'

'How about in yourself . . . how are you feeling?'

He looks away. Looks back at me. 'It's rough.'

'It sounds rough.'

He smiles.

'Okay,' I say. 'Let's talk to your oncologist about your pain medication. And we'll get you something stronger for the nausea. What else can we do to help, Richard?'

At the end of the three months, almost as if heaven and angels exist, one of our work team hands in her resignation and I'm offered a permanent full-time position and I take it without hesitation and for a further six months I work hard and practice yoga and visit Winsome once a week and life smooths out like an estuary nearing the sea.

'It's such a god damn relief,' I say to Winsome, breathing so deep and fast I'm dizzy, 'to be financially responsible. I think being reliant on the government for a fortnightly pittance – sickness benefit, disability support – is also a kind of straightjacket. Like being hospitalised and medicated and told you're not . . . you're just not . . .'

'I see that,' Winsome says, quietly. 'But you're making wonderful progress. It's a delight to see.'

'Really?'

'Yes. Really.'

'Thank you, Winsome. That means . . .'

real connection kind of love gratefulness smallness strength hope

'. . . that means a lot.'

Richard has come into hospital by ambulance with a bowel obstruction. I go up to the oncology ward to see him.

'Dr T and I had the big talk,' Richard says. 'To keep going with the chemo . . . or not. I've decided not.'

'Okay,' I say. And then I get up from the chair and kneel down next to the bed so our eyes are at the same level and I hold his thin, dry hand. 'Bloody hard decision.'

He huffs, grins, frowns. There are tears in his eyes.

'So. This is it,' he says.

'Is your family here?' I ask.

'Yeah, they've gone to get me some stuff from home. They'll be back.'

'Good.'

'I've been wondering . . . what happens now?'

'Do you mean about palliative care?'

'Yes. And about . . . you know . . .'

'About dying?'

'Yes.'

I nod, hold his hand. There are tears in his eyes.

'At night I keep thinking . . .' he says.

'Ah huh?'

'How do you die?' he asks. 'I mean . . . how do you actually . . . die?'

I take a breath and think about how to reply. I want to be honest. I don't want to scare him. I'm scared that he'll see I'm scared (to talk honestly about dying to a man who is dying).

'I can talk with you from my knowledge and experience Richard, but I don't know everything – far from it – and I might be wrong. I mean there are only a few set truths and so much of what happens will be very personal to you . . . okay?'

'Please . . .'

'First, there's a physical process . . . of the body slowing down and then shutting down. So people usually rest more and sleep more and more and often don't feel hungry. And then you may have times of not being conscious to most things, but you may still hear music and the voices of people talking with you. Your breathing changes, it may get faster for a time and then much slower. Sometimes people feel restless and sometimes people wake up for a while and then fall back into a very deep sleep. The right medication for pain and for feeling restless is so important and the palliative care team will make sure of that.'

We sit in silence for a few minutes.

'You know,' I say quietly. 'Whatever is important to you, whatever is sacred, whatever feels right for you and your family . . . so long as you are comfortable in your body . . . there aren't any rules.'

We sit in silence, holding hands.

Then he says thanks and I squeeze his hands and go back to the stairs and whisper, oh fuck, with each step down, tears blurring the stairs and stairwell and the people striding past with purpose, on and up.

21

One day, walking down a quiet street with a park at the end of it, I pass an apartment for sale that is open – right now – for inspection. I go in. The main bedroom upstairs has large windows overlooking mature oak and silver birch trees. The kitchen is old and the carpet is bile-green shag but the living area is big enough for books and music with adequate wall space for etchings and linocuts, posters and paintings and photographs. There's a spare bedroom for friends and a separate toilet and a courtyard with high walls covered in ivy.

I turn up to the auction alone, wearing old track-pants and a bright orange, crocheted beanie. At the end of the auction the apartment is passed in, but I'm the highest bidder so we enter 'negotiations.' The estate agent trips back and forth between the owners and me.

'You must be so nervous!' she says, standing well inside my personal space, breathing fast. 'I'm nervous, and it's not even going to be my new home.'

I frown.

She smiles, red lips and teeth.

'There are more important things,' I say.

She frowns.

I sniff.

After half an hour, the owners agree to my price, which is actually my parents' price. Though I've saved enough to pay the deposit on the mortgage, they are financial guarantors and without their support I couldn't afford anything like this place.

My father builds a red gum bookcase that spans nearly the length and height of the living room. It is the centrepiece of the apartment. The cats stalk through the new rooms like they're prowling in the jungle. At the end of each day I ask what it is they have discovered. We all sleep on the big bed with the windows wide open to the air and the darkness and the creeping of the ivy and the brimming silver birches.

'I've booked a flight to New York,' I say to Zoë one Sunday evening, sitting in the courtyard, watching the light fade, artery to vein.

'What?'

'Manhattan, Queens—'

'Duh. I do know that. Are you manic?'

'I am not.'

'Have you told Winsome?'

'She's cautiously positive.'

'Why now?'

'I've been thinking that I might always have a fits and starts kind of life. Able, unable. Sick, well,' I lean forward, clasp my hands. 'I'd like the well bits to be meaningful, I'd like to experience stuff and explore, meet people, learn. Manage better.'

Zoë nods but she doesn't look convinced. 'I get that,' she says. 'And New York sounds . . . fantastic, bloody hell, it really does,

142

but . . . I dunno . . . have you thought it through?'

'Yes.'

'Have you?'

'Yes.'

Of course I have. The Met! The Guggenheim, Central Park! The world.

Zoë tips her head to the right. Her eyes search for mine.

Oh. Now I get it.

'Oh,' I say.

'You bought this flat, what . . . three months ago?'

'Yeah,' I say. 'But I've saved hard for this. The mortgage isn't going anywhere.'

Zoë crosses her legs, uncrosses them. Crosses them. Looks at me.

I have not thought this through. It was so clear and so right a minute ago. So easy.

I close my eyes. 'I'm such a stupid fuck.'

'Hey?'

'Me.'

'I'm not saying give it up, I'm saying be careful. I mean . . . be careful with your money. And think about what could happen if you don't get enough sleep over there, or you get mega-obsessed with something.'

'Yeah. You're right. You're just like Winsome. Too bloody rational. But thanks Zo. God. Seriously. Thanks.'

'Take your meds.'

'Every single morning and every single night.'

'No exceptions.'

'No exceptions.'

'And for God's sake don't take too much spending money!'

I laugh.

'And call me or call Winsome if you think you're not doing well.'

'Thanks, honey.'

'I mean it.'

We smile at each other across the fur of sleeping cats.

22

JFK airport to Greenpoint, Brooklyn requires an Air Train ride followed by the A Subway and then the G Subway to Nassau Avenue. It's ten at night and I'm on the other side of the world. I have my backpack and map and a bottle of water and I'm on the other side of the world.

Rising up from the subway rubbish bags and piles of newspapers tied with string line Manhattan Avenue. All the shops are Polish. Most are closed but the bottle shop is open and I buy a bottle of vodka. I find my hostel and sit for a long time on the bed, sipping the vodka, letting it roar in my mouth and throat. Then I take the lithium tablets, the venlafaxine and a lorazepam and turn on the black and white television and doze.

At 5 a.m. I walk across the street past the NYPD depot to a bakery whose window is a tender yellow glow in the early morning dark. Inside are rows of glazed doughnuts filled with rose petal jam, babka, all sorts of *chruściki* (angel's wings) and ah, coffee. I walk back down into the warm subterranean world of the subway, resurface by Brooklyn Bridge.

Between the two stone towers of Brooklyn Bridge is the steel frame, functional below my feet, in perfect symmetry above them. The bridge has an energy to it – the lights and the cars and its own singular beauty. I take giant steps, up on my toes, grinning, breathing. The sun is rising behind me, throwing itself at the East River, reflecting there and rising again . . .

Down in Battery Park the street vendors are setting up their vans. I ask for a hot dog with mustard and onions, chilli and sauerkraut.

'Brilliant morning,' I say to the vendor. He doesn't look at me and he doesn't reply, just stretches out his arm with the hot dog wrapped in a white serviette like he's stopping traffic. I walk north along Trinity Place and think of Berenice Abbott's black and white photographs of Manhattan. She used a Century Universal eight by ten camera that concertina-like, could almost see around corners. Berenice said of New York that, 'its tempo is like the tempo of the compressed air drill'.

Oh yes.

I mutter as I walk – about light and shadow. I mutter about angle and perspective and depth, but none of my digital photos are anything like Berenice's, which leaves me feeling exhilarated and anguished in equal measure. She had such a fine eye for . . . the liquid of time.

Back up Broadway I go inside a cafe and ask for a double shot skinny flat white.

'Excuse me?' say both young men behind the counter at the same time.

I repeat.

Silence.

Horror. No espresso machine. It starts to rain, fine as silk thread. I walk north on Lafayette Street looking for coffee but the intricacy of the buildings keeps my eyes skyward. On the corner of East 12th and Broadway is the eighteen miles of books that comprise the Strand Bookstore. Four stories of new books, second-hand and rare books and a decent amount of stuff first written in a language other than English.

MADNESS

I find the second-hand poetry. I love the musty smell, the yellow-brown pages, the crookedly underlined passages, the notes – things someone, who is otherwise invisible to me, found significant or erudite or beautiful, and so we make a kind of secret connection through the medium of William Carlos Williams. 'Icarus drowning' is underlined twice in dark blue ink, marking the paper so deeply I have to stop suddenly on the stairs. Outside again and the sky is colourless between the glazed terracotta and limestone buildings. I take the subway to the corner of Central Park.

ha ha ha ha ha ha ha get down on the ground bitch ha ha on the ground

They're screaming.

I kneel on the grass under a sugar maple in the park. Cover my ears.

Screaming, my head beating like a heart.

on the ground vile ha ha ha ha ha on the ground vile do it do it

Fold myself up, eyes shut, body shut. Eyelids pricked by the ends of the grass.

we're here to kill you ha ha bitch on the ground vile do it do it

It is dusk when it stops. Softer light. My legs from thighs to toes are numb and blue and above is the sugar maple, roaring colour, and I use its leaves as a visual anaesthetic while I stretch out and wait for the painful tingling and rush of blood. The dizziness clears quicker on standing the second time. The sky is the hue of skin, flushed.

I take the subway back to Greenpoint and get into the narrow bed, under the chrysanthemum doona and I drown the people in my head with earphones up loud and vodka and they leave me alone and I sleep until four in the morning, at which time I wander the nearby brownstone streets until the Polish bakery opens and I sit drinking coffee, re-writing sentences and swinging around on the chair, watching the light change from grey to vanilla and finally, reluctantly, I see that I'm unable to capture the all-five-senses, unabridged feel of New York City in words. I take the subway to West 53rd Street – to the Museum of Modern Art.

'But perhaps my art is the art of a lunatic,' Marc Chagall said, and I wonder about this, standing in front of his *I and the Village*, painting number 1335. The green-faced peasant with his moonlight lips, the goat (or cow? lamb?), the fractured perspective, the eyes – one black on white, the other white on black – holding each other like hands, and then the circles, the sun and the moon and the earth. It is unorthodox, magical, non-sequential, imbued with multiple and even conflicting emotions. I stand in front of *I and the Village* for a very long time, run my palms over my eyes when they're wet.

'That is so not the point,' says a young girl sitting near me, talking on her pink mobile. 'I never said that. Who told you? I'm gonna break his arse. I know. I KNOW. Oh my God.' She stands up. 'There goes my fucking hero, watch him as he burns. Huh? Dave Grohl, you doorknob.' She laughs, and I laugh and catch a bus past Cartier and Saks and get off near Bryant Park with its wooden seats and plane trees and view over the tops of the trees to the Chrysler Building – all silver in the sun. Gertrude Stein in bronze sits cross-legged, her hands relaxed and unfurled in her lap. She's brooding or thinking or imagining, or perhaps all three at once.

ha ha ha ha ha ha ha get down on the ground you bitch ha ha on the ground

They're screaming.

I kneel on the gravel. Cover my ears.

Screaming.

on the ground vile ha ha ha ha ha ha on the ground do it do it VILE

I fold myself up, forehead on the gravel, eyes shut. There's not enough room for my lungs. But after a minute, a part of me, somewhere inside, shouts, 'Get up. Fucking get up.' And I do, and once my pupils shrink back in the light, here are other people walking and people sitting talking and drinking coffee from paper cups with little rivulets and they look relaxed, unconcerned. No one else is curled up on the ground.

on the ground vile ha ha ha ha ha ha on the ground

I look up at the American Standard Building with its solid black brick façade and terracotta friezes coated in gold. I look around again at the other people in the park and at Gertrude Stein's serene face. I pick up my backpack and walk north on Sixth Avenue. The streetlights are coming on.

vile ha ha ha ha ha

'Piss. Off,' I whisper, in time with my feet, following a line of yellow taxies to Times Square.

'You fuckers,' I whisper, and then a bit louder, 'PISS. OFF.'

It must be like standing up to an abuser for the very first time: terrifying and a tiny bit thrilling.

Just south of Times Square, someone is standing under a streetlight preaching. I walk nearer and take out a notebook and pen. He has two men close on either side of him and two behind, all wearing silver chains and bandanas, one holding an open bible. The preacher is wrapped in a tunic the colour of ripe tomatoes, around his waist is a bright gold belt like he's just won a heavy weight boxing title. 'I say to you! Woe to the shepherds of Yisra'el! We are like sheep that have gone astray!' He's on the tips of his toes. 'For the life of the flesh is in the blood and God has given it to us to make atonement for our souls!' He pauses rather dramatically and stares at the little crowd of people around him. 'For it is only the blood that makes atonement for the soul.'

This is a curious sermon. For it is only blood that makes atonement for the soul. I walk on and try to make sense of it, because it is close to my own philosophy when I am depressed. But do we mean the same thing?

My new hostel for the final of four weeks is on Eighth Avenue, Chelsea, next to an erotica store for men who love other men. In the window of the store are some sexy mannequins, one with a patent leather jock strap, one with nipple clamps, another with a fabulous-looking harness in black and red. There are pumps and pouches and rings and mesh and fishnet. Steam is rising from the underground Con Edison pipes.

Out the back of the main hostel building is a sunken courtyard with a wooden table running down the centre and sitting around the table are young Hispanic men in shorts and singlets drinking beer. All of them are ripped. I can see how beautifully the deltoid muscle of the shoulder inserts itself between the heads of triceps and biceps in the upper arm and how pectoralis major is like an open fan over the chest wall and the perfect contour of brachioradialis around the elbow. I slide off my backpack and sit on the steps leading down to the courtyard and get out a book and pretend to read.

The women's dorm has six bunks. Tonight it's Maricela from Bogotá, Marie-Anne from Paris, Aisha and Jac from Saskatchewan, and me. Aisha has her hair in cornrows running side-to-side and then extending from the base of her skull almost to her waist.

'How long did it take to braid?' I ask Aisha.

'Eight hours,' she says. 'Over two days.'

'Fabuleuse!' says Marie-Anne.

We swap little shots of information about our lives. I offer the vodka. We laugh. Here I am on the other side of the world, a normal young woman visiting New York City for the first time, warm and alive and with a mind of her own.

In the morning I catch a bus to the Metropolitan Museum of Art. I have a map of the main building with its two million works of art spanning five thousand years. Greek and Roman Art to the left, Egyptian to the right, European Sculpture straight ahead and another world above. I sit down. The echo of voices in the Great Hall rolls over me. I'm under a waterfall of stimuli. The water is heavy. There's a rush of noise, a wave, and then silence.

'Excuse me, Ma'am . . .'

The voice: so close, I shatter.

'Ma'am? Are you okay?'

I grope . . . gather the shards.

'Oh yes,' I say. 'Yes, fine, sorry. Sorry.'

'You've been sitting here an awful long time. Do you need help?'

'Not at all, thank you, sorry, um . . .' I stand and smile. The woman smiles. We walk together toward the main exit.

'Have you enjoyed the exhibitions?' she asks, pleasantly.

'Very much indeed.'

Central Park in the late evening is quiet. Few people. Balls of light along the paths – white light and yellow, picking up the tree branches and throwing shadow. Piles of autumn leaves. The sky a murky orange where the encompassing Manhattan lights are sopped up by clouds. It is cold and I walk briskly, thinking about religion. It's not belief in one particular god that I'm drawn to; rather it is the broader concept of faith and derived from it, meaning. I'm curious about anyone who is sure that the path he or she is taking through life is somehow intrinsically *the right one*. What is it like to be part of such a community, to be committed to it, to be guided by it, to have respect for it, to yearn for its growth, to wake every morning with a sense of purpose?

There is a group of trees to my left covered in fairy lights and I take off my glasses so that the pinpoints of light refract, and then I fall without warning onto a hip-high barbwire fence. The pain in my right groin is so sudden and fierce that I roll off the fence to the ground and wonder if I've pierced my femoral artery. I lie on my back on the damp grass, looking up at the trees with their tiny lights and at the near-by hedges cut into animals. A fine rain starts to fall and it occurs to me, much like an epiphany, that I don't want to die here.

Inevitably the pain eases and of course I haven't pierced my femoral artery, but I lie with the lights and the hedges and the realisation that I'd really seriously like to stay alive. The people in my head laugh but I don't mind. In the rain, the sky and the stars are streaming.

On the plane home, squashed into cattle class between two middle-aged businessmen and the presents for friends and family at my feet, through all twenty hours, I chew over the links between spirit and faith and melancholic illness. Is the 'illness' a response to meaninglessness? Is it a somewhat illogical response to a spiritual void, a lonely soul? And therefore could a cure be prescribed *not as a drug*, but *by a particular physical and spiritual environment*? Suddenly it all makes sense. New York City is my cure!

God almighty.

Yes.

'Coffee,' I say to the flight attendant. 'Two cups, with sugar, please.'

Yes.

With New York City as my cure, I can finally get off the psychotropic drugs. To absorb the world purely, to absorb New York City and let it heal, I must surely be free from the interference of mind-altering substances like lithium and the anti-psychotics and the anti-depressants.

Taking lithium is like wearing a particular kind of blinkers. Lithium curbs creativity. It blocks the ability to make unique connections between objects and concepts. It blunts the acuteness of sensitivity to words and sound and colour. It stunts passion. I remember friend and poet N.O.'s slam poem about her own psychotropic medication:

> Can't really do work on it,
> Can't really talk on it,
> Never can drink on it,
> Can't really drive on it,
> Can't get a job on it,
> Can't really read on it,
> Can't remember much on it,
> Can't enjoy sex on it,
> Certainly can't have a baby on it.

And British psychiatrist R.D. Laing wrote, 'The cracked mind of the schizophrenic may let in light which does not enter the intact minds of many sane people whose minds are closed.'

I don't have schizophrenia, but lithium does hinder the letting in of light and perhaps even (in the words of an Chassidic Rabbi), *l'havi or l'olam* – the bringing of light into the world.

Seven hours of rumination and I'm sure. Before we descend into Melbourne I empty the bottle of lithium tablets into the aeroplane toilet. Gush and suck and gone.

23

November, the end of spring. The air is slowly warmer and the dark is picking up energy. I haven't taken lithium for three weeks. The last of the magnolias are flowering and I'm in front of them like my shoes have been glued to the ground because of palpitations.

The beauty of ordinary life.

One Saturday Zoë comes over for dinner.

'Why are your clothes drying all over the chairs?' she asks.

'It's the clotheshorse. There's something about its shape – it's like a carcass. I'm not sure . . . I just have this really strong sense that it's leering. All that wire . . . you know?'

'Not really, no. Are you okay?'

'Will be once I get rid of the clotheshorse.'

I haven't taken any lithium for seven weeks, and today I understand why the minor key is sadder than the major. The interval of a Minor Third (three semitones) mirrors the expression of sadness in human speech and is the change in pitch of emergency sirens. The evenings, the nights are when the minor third clutches me in its slow and melancholic way – clutches and holds. By morning my heart has doubled in weight. It is there in the centre of my chest cavity, this dense red muscle that clenches blood of its own accord, throbbing – lubdub – with portent. I carry it around with me and size up its heaviness and its meaning. In the day I'm suddenly afraid of the omnipotence of sunlight, of its ability to make me visible. Melancholia is stretching her generous wings.

I wear the burnt orange beanie with the holes in it where the wool is unravelling, and long skirts over long pants and boots and jumpers and coats. The dark is picking up energy. The doves on Fitzroy Street worry me. How do I keep them from dying?

On my lunch break from work I walk around the city buying copies of the same edition of *The Big Issue* from as many vendors as I can find. Air tunnels up Flinders Lane and hurts the epidermis – the outer layer of my skin. The sound of cars on the road scratches my inner ears – the labyrinths, the cochlear and the oh-so-fine hair cells. Sunlight falls on my retinae – hits the rods and cones – shivers them. The leaves on the plane trees are brutal-green.

By the time I'm back at my desk I'm wet with sweat and my legs are heavy.

'Kate, it's nearly summer and you're dressed for the arctic,' says one of my colleagues.

'I'm cold-blooded,' I say.

She looks confused. 'Are you okay?'

spawn death you spawn death

They've subjected me to an electric current. Their voices are sudden knives. I start to shake – a fine, full-body tremor.

'Sure, just cold.'

death you spawn death

I try to hold on to sanity by falling deep into fictional worlds, falling in deep, staying under for as long as I can hold my breath. I read in the morning, on the train, in my lunch break at work, all evening, through the ink-blue-black of half the night. I'm reading a book a day swallowing the characters whole.

you spawn death spawn death is gathering

Around my neck is a replica Athenian coin on a silver chain. The head of Athena goddess of wisdom, goddess of war, is on one side and there's an owl on the other. Owls are also symbols of wisdom – and of dread. Wherever I go, I hold in my right hand two card-sized black and white engravings by Albrecht Dürer. They lie next to my pillow at night.

death is gathering

I start drinking.

Whisky, red wine, anything to shut them up.

I cancel my appointment with Winsome via email. If my heart were now removed and weighed against the feather of Ma'at, it would be devoured by the part-lion, part-crocodile beast guarding a path to the afterlife. Winsome is decent and principled. What if my dark leaky heart is contagious? What if I spawn death?

On the train are school kids laughing and whispering about kissing and adults who are tired and normal or bored and normal or intent on one another and normal. The seats are too narrow, I'm terrified of my neighbour's skin, the air is stiff; thick and hot and stiff, my eyes are all pupil in spite of the sunlight. The graffiti on the walls beside the train line is significant but I don't know how to unravel its meaning. VOID MEOW BIG! OH YEAH! PUNK<<<MANIACS MOKE BUZZ COCKED. Blood is running down the windows.

Once or twice a day I go into the women's toilets, into the farthest cubicle from the door and curl up on the floor next to the sanitary bin and close my eyes and I don't move for thirty or forty minutes. After eight or nine hours of desperate normality at work I'm completely unnerved by the thought of other commuters standing so close with so much flesh. I pay a hefty fee for taxies home.

This particular evening the moon in its thin crescent phase; the dark side just visible by earthshine, thus transforming the whole from a part-circle into an animate sphere, a pockmarked eye. It takes forever to walk up the driveway and my keys are heavy and once inside the house I feed the cats and take my shoes off and get into bed. There's a shard of sunlight breaching the closed curtains, but I'm not moving now. No poetry, no television, no telephone, no further light. I have a mixed CD of Lisa Gerrard and Jeff Buckley. I play it on repeat. If the music were translated into colour, it would be black and the grey of a post-apocalyptic wasteland. Each night, in a tiny dinghy far out to sea, out in the ocean with oceany waves and an oceany swell, I fall into deep troughs, so deep that inside them, I cannot see the sky.

'Hush,' I whisper to the cats. 'Hush.'

The heaviness in the centre of my chest makes it hard to breathe. Air is full of chlorine. One morning The Presence takes up residence over my left shoulder. He is an amorphous mass; squat and angry and bitter. He leers and mutters in a strangely breathy way. To soften His voice I drive out to the big, generic GP clinics in the suburbs and ask for drugs – benzos if I can get them or tramadol, even codeine. As the days pass I make a new CD of four Jeff Buckley songs and listen to that on repeat. Then only one song, Leonard Cohen's 'Halleluiah', over and over and over. Curled up. Tight.

At work I file manila folders neatly and delete old emails, shred personal documents, clean my desk with disinfectant and arrange some annual leave. The backs of my hands and my arms are a repeatedly curious maze of black ink lines and swirls, vaguely Celtic.

'Are you all right?' my manager asks.

death you spawn death

'I'm sorry,' I say. 'Just really tired. Possibly a virus.'

When all music spikes my insides I put on the BBC World Service and the English version of Radio Deutsche Welle. When English hurts – the words, the meaning – I listen half the night to SBS Radio broadcasting in Portuguese and Cambodian, Croatian and Arabic, drinking whisky straight from the bottle.

They're coming through the phone now, hissing—

you are stench stench

you spawn unclean and evil

death you spawn death

Or sometimes they just laugh, high and mirthless.

I stop showering because The Presence is a voyeur – an enormous, predatory voyeur. I stop eating because I have no appetite and everything tastes like newspaper. I read and write scratchy sentences and drink whisky until the clutch and suck of Him ebbs. My house is filthy. I am filthy, my hair and clothes unwashed, my breath ketotic. The fridge is empty, there are piles of rubbish in the hallway, my body smells, my bed smells. Amongst a pile of CDs on my living room floor I discover Max Bruch's *Kol Nidrei*. It is an Italian recording; the soloist accompanied by eight other cellos. I play it on repeat all through the night. Kol Nidre: All Vows, the prayer of erev Yom Kippur. All vows . . . atonement. Atonement . . . death.

spawn you are stench you are spawn death WE SAID (shouting) *you spawn death*

Words are pressing in on my head and eyes. There are lumpy

bruises on my arms – my wrists, my forearms, and welts where I have scratched at my skin in the night. Deborah rings and Zoë rings and my parents ring.

'Are you okay?' they ask.

'Really, I'm okay.'

'Are you safe?'

'Quite safe.'

death is gathering

In the night, the sensual night, the million-star-spawning-night. I wait. Avē Marīa, sancta Marīa, hail hail—the night offers communion, but He is here, heavy on my shoulder, whispering His darling doctrine in my left ear with breath like thick fog. He is a hangman's noose around my neck. I write about the squashed arteries, the cervical fracture, the stoppered trachea, the tongue, the terminal erection. And then the nakedness on stainless steel; body stripped back bare as that of a newborn. Carbon leaving earth in a dream.

24

Winsome rings and suggests, firmly, that I make an appointment.

'Not okay,' I say eventually, hunched up on her couch in long pants, a skirt, jumper, winter coat and high black boots.

Winsome looks at me calmly.

Dead self. Sitting here. In this chair. The relief.

'What's happening?' Winsome asks.

Can't face her eyes. Him.

'All this shit,' I say, monotone.

unclean spawn

'In notebooks. That I've written in the night.'

My handwriting is not mine. It is His. I hold the pen in my hand but the words that form on the page are His.

Winsome is very still.

Dead self. Old bone. Him.

'It doesn't make sense. None at all.'

'What else is happening?' Winsome asks.

unclean and evil devil and spawn

'The phone,' I say.

Can't feel the air.

'Nowhere is safe,' I say.

Winsome waits.

Silence for a minute outside my head.

'The melancholia of Dürer's engraving,' I say.

'Meaning . . .?' asks Winsome.

'I don't know how to get rid of it.'

Talk to the floor. Can't face her eyes. Him.

'Get rid of the melancholia?' she asks.

'Dead self.'

evil devil spawn you are stench you are spawn death WE SAID (shouting) *you spawn death*

Unwind off the couch. Slow old bone.

Scrunch on the floor.

Winsome watches but she doesn't comment. Then she says, 'There have been times when you have been in a better space: aware of your feelings, finding pleasure in your surroundings and senses. At present, however, you seem to be in a very different place.'

Nod.

'I appreciate that you are not in the frame of mind for therapy. I'd like you to make an urgent appointment with Aaron. It's essential, Kate, that you and he discuss medication.'

Hunch down.

Whisper, 'Narcotics cannot still the tooth that nibbles at the soul.'

'If I can make an appointment for today or tomorrow will you go?' Winsome asks.

Nod.

Aaron listens to me stutter for ten minutes and then he says, 'Hospital.'

Everyone smokes in the inpatient unit. Tobacco is currency. There's another new patient on the ward today, pacing and smoking rollies in the courtyard. That singular-psychosis-energy is streaming from his skin, his feet, his arms, his eyes. His eyes are black diamonds – the glint and flint – it is rare, like rare meat, all the juice and flair. His stare enters me through my eyes and exits through the occipital lobe at the back of my head.

'Kate! Move away please.' One of the nurses wanders over. 'Move away.'

I do.

For the first two days in hospital I don't get out of bed even for my bladder and staff leave me alone. Then they must have decided that the only way to get me up in the morning is to come into the bedroom in pairs, as loudly as possible, open the curtains, peel the blankets and sheets off me and say, 'We're not leaving, Kate, until you are out of bed.'

'There isn't a single, plausible reason for moving,' I say, eyes closed. My voice makes me want to vomit.

'Gorgeous day,' says Damien, my regular contact nurse. 'Blue sky.'

beware we said devil we said hang your hair right there

'Come on please. Now.'

'I need a forklift.'

Damien laughs. But I am serious. What's left of the body is already dead.

When I finally lumber into the communal area, the largest person I've ever seen is sitting at one of the tables eating cornflakes. He takes the lid off the plastic sugar pot and pours sugar like a waterfall into his bowl. He sits to the side of the table because his belly won't fit underneath. His legs are wide apart and I can see his penis through the taut gaps between the buttons of his pyjama fly.

In the courtyard I sit on the wooden bench with my notebooks and bag of other books and stare for a long time at the brown concrete tiles.

unclean and evil devil spawn you are stench you are spawn death you spawn death you spawn death

'Kate?' says Damien from the doorway. 'Aaron's ready to see you.'

As we go through the community area, a young man comes out of HDU holding a young woman's hand, with one of the nursing staff on his other side. I know him – James and I were in a uni class together a few years ago. He looks at me without recognition, shoots out his left hand and grips my arm.

'They're trying to steal my logic,' he says, low and fast. 'They're a security company disguised as a hospital and they're contravening the Universal Declaration of Human Rights.'

I don't say anything.

'They administer harmful substances!' his voice rises as the nurse tries to walk him away. 'We're lab rats! They track and trace us with satellites. Ask them to reverse their smiles because it's false advertising.'

'Oh James,' says the young woman. She strokes his head.

'Don't,' he says.

Her eyes fill with tears.

'Tell them lies; otherwise they'll rip off your identity!' he shouts at the roof.

Damien and I walk into the interview room. Aaron is already here with my medical record open in front of him.

'How are you today?' Aaron asks.

'Breathing.'

Aaron suppresses a yawn.

'Come on Kate, you can do better than that,' says Damien.

I stare at the floor. 'It has been decreed.'

'What has been decreed?'

'My death.'

'Oh.'

I nod.

'Are you sure?' asks Damien.

I give him all of my eyes – right through, cornea to retina, right through.

In the corner of the room, Lily is on the floor in her crib. Lily was born different. Her neck repulses her head. Her tongue sticks straight out, writhing like a pale eel. Lily's eyes are bent sideways; part blue, part green. Separate from one another. Alone in their sockets. She keens all through the night, flails arms and legs, forms positions unholy for a child. Hair smothers her crown and brow; not even the sides of her face are delicious to touch. Adults sometimes look kindly– attempt embrace, but Lily makes a bridge of her spine so high she might as well be boneless. Perhaps she is. Her hands are always fists.

How do I articulate Lily to these two neat, clean men? The connection between my brain and mouth is blocked, stoppered or perhaps severed. I sit there with the pain – the visceral pain, centred in the chest, heavy as plutonium and glacier-cold. And the soul-pain, because the very essence of self is damaged and damaging. Then there is the mind, tunnelling itself straight to hell. I can't articulate this. I sit there.

Later I walk back into the courtyard because I'm not allowed in my room and the television is on in the community area. The television impregnates: it is too loud and too fast and too bright. Naava is playing the ward's acoustic guitar. She plays intimately; a few people gather round to listen. Two patients are kissing on a bench, her legs in between his legs, her hands, his hands, feeling their way over each other's skin, lips. They glow a little.

'Close your eyes,' she says to him. 'Go on.' He does. Then she says, 'I love you I love you I love you I love you.'

Naava plays 'Blues run the game' by Nick Drake, quietly and

perfectly. The music heals one of the broken things inside me. When she finishes, Andrew and I clap.

'There's never going to be a Second Coming,' says Andrew, his eyes suddenly red and bright.

Damien says, 'Kate, let's have a chat.'

In my room I curl up on the bed and Damien sits opposite on one of those generic, plastic hospital chairs.

'How's it going?' he asks.

'If you put me in a brown cardboard box and taped it up and walked away, I wouldn't care.'

'When was the last time you had a shower?'

'Ah . . . well, the thing is . . .'

'Yes?'

'A month ago. I think. I don't remember.'

'When was the last time you changed your clothes?'

I don't know the answer.

'Your clothes smell awful.'

'It's . . . I can't . . .' I hold my breath all the way in.

He waits.

'It's not just me in the shower, that's the problem.'

'I don't understand.'

'. . . there's Him.'

'Who?'

'Shit.' I stare up at the sprinkler outlets, metal flowers, in the ceiling.

'Nothing up there is going to help you, Kate.'

'I call Him The Presence, okay, He's here, He's always here, He doesn't leave me the fuck alone, He whispers in my left ear on and on and on, I don't know why He's here, I didn't bloody well invite Him and I'd quite like to kill Him, all right, so now you know, you can go ahead and lock me up.'

'Thank you for being so honest. Can I talk to your doctor about this?'

'Oh so he can lock me up. Brilliant. No, okay, yes, okay.'

'You're shaking.'

'Well it's not every day you get to admit that you're mad.'

'Mad?'

'Yes, you know, loony, batty, bonkers, completely fucked in the head.'

'Is that what you are?'

'Yes.'

'I don't think so. Part of your brain is not working properly, but we can treat that. That's why you're here.'

I roll my eyes. Damien is looking at me directly; his eyes are brown and clear and appear to be emitting their own light from somewhere deep inside him.

'Okay,' I say.

'We gave you a series of psychometric tests when you were here a couple of years ago. Do you remember?' he asks.

'No.'

'Well your visual and verbal responses and your processing speed were off the charts.'

I stare at my knees.

'There is a link between creativity and some kinds of mental illness.'

'I've read about it.'

'Many people in the creative arts are affected in one way or another, usually with one or more episodes of depression or hypomania. And about half have a problematic relationship with alcohol and/or other drugs at some time in their lives.'

I smile at my knees, 'I've got the second part.'

166

'I really do want to help you, while you're here. Will you work with me?' His voice is soft and warm.

The people in my head cackle.

'I'm a persistent vegetable, a breathing, shitting shell. I kneel in my swill.'

'That's the illness talking. Your life is before you. We can get you through this rough patch and I'd like to start by asking you to come and see us whenever it gets particularly bad.'

Nothing about this conversation amounts to anything, but I appreciate that Damien has taken the time to bother with it, so I say, 'Okay. Thanks Damien,' and I walk into the courtyard and here's Max, shuffling towards me. He's about seventy, very thin, elegantly dressed, coiffed hair. When he opens his mouth his two teeth are yellow and black and his breath is a fetid mix of cigarettes, pus and acetone. He stands in front of me, where I'm sitting cross-legged on one of the wooden benches.

'Look at you!' he shouts. 'You're a fucking dirty bitch prostitute! How much do you charge?'

I look at him.

'You dirty bitch! Are you soliciting me? I'm calling the police! Hey! She's a prostitute! Hey! I've got five dollars.'

I just look.

'Bitch, you dirty bitch,' he says. 'Hey! There's a fucking prostitute here!' And then he spits a thick, yellow gob onto the ground in front of me. It bubbles, and he shuffles away, stopping every two steps to hold up his hands, glaring, mouthing 'dirty bitch'.

The newspaper is here and I copy out my horoscope:

Your planet Mercury makes a harmonious link to Pluto, so today is one of those days when you'll probably feel all your brain cogs are superbly well-oiled. It is a perfect opportunity for making plans or analysing crucial issues. Enjoy the light and positive feeling that comes with both heart and mind working smoothly and astutely. Favourable colours are pink and parchment.

Then I go inside and write—

the life that was once ~~much~~ balls of cells burning sugar and green mitochondria, ~~swum~~ swirling and sweeping and bumping into ~~one another~~ one another is no longer conscious. No touch no warmth from the blanket that covers this thing—this terrifying frame. The flowers ~~wilt~~ at the bed end wilt droop lower hang their old slow heads. Tulips mauve and pink..

There are no easy deaths.
There is no sweet repose.   I've tried the grog, the creamy alcoholic haze and ~~from my darkest find love~~
I couldn't find love.

Naava and I are now sharing a room.

'Hi, I'm Naava,' she says every morning. 'When were you admitted?'

'Hi Naava. I've been here a couple of weeks.'

'Really? Have we met before?'

'Yeah.'

'Shit.'

'It's okay, it's the ECT you're having. It fucks up your memory.'

'Does it?'

'Yes.'

She says something in Hebrew that I don't understand. She has pale skin, very dark hair, immensely intelligent eyes and like Brett, she looks as lost as someone who finds herself in the middle of an unexpected dream. We talk about music – PJ Harvey and Broken Social Scene. Our despair matches.

In the afternoon James is released from HDU and walks through the ward into the courtyard as if completely new to the world. I remember him when we were at uni together – then, as now, he was passionate and articulate and creative. Then, as now, he wrote nihilistic poetry. He wore pants and shirts and jewellery in a myriad of styles and fabrics and somehow made the whole thing look like a cutting edge outfit. Back then he had his own interior design business. I don't ask him about it.

'They said I was making up things about their coffee,' he says, as we sit together, drinking coffee. The tiles are hot under my buttocks and bare feet.

'They're scared of people like me and you who have ideas and create new thoughts. They arrest us because they want our knowledge and then they torture us.' He stands up suddenly, dropping his coffee. He looks at the sky, 'Criminals have more rights.'

Hot coffee is all over my face and arms and legs but I don't move.

'If you tell the straight truth,' he says, sitting down again, 'if you say, hey what the hell are you doing with your life, or if you say, hey, psychiatry is a theatre of cruelty, they can't bear it because it diminishes their power. That's when they start their experiments.'

As an inpatient I'm prescribed an interesting cocktail of medication: olanzapine, mirtazapine, lithium, periodic chlorpromazine and periodic diazepam. It is in one sense effective: I'm so sedated, so completely unable to think, so emotionally and physically numb, that The Presence's talons shrink down into matchsticks.

Friends from work, Bev and Chris and Monique visit, Zoë and Tanya and my parents visit, and I sit with them on the green vinyl couches and I'm only partially aware of their physical presence. I'm not asleep, neither am I awake.

Damien lends me some books by writers he admires. There are letters on the pages. I don't know how to turn them into words. We talk about making small, daily steps towards improving my mental state. He cajoles me out of bed in the morning for a walk in the park. Here are the oak trees – their branches like arms lending out scraps of nirvana where the sun touches the leaves.

We talk about hope. He has a kind of extraordinary faith that I'll recover, and as I do get better, I hold onto it too, like we are together clutching the string of a balloon.

Sometimes in the night I ring Aaron's rooms and recite Arthur Rimbaud into his answering machine:

Je regrette les temps où la sève du monde,
L'eau du fleuve, le sang rose des arbres verts,
Dans les veines de Pan mettaient un univers!
(. . . in the veins of Pan, a whole universe!)

'Come on,' says Josie, my allocated nurse for the morning. 'Shower.'

I take off my clothes and turn the water on and stand under it. I cannot touch my body. I stand for a reasonable number of minutes, turn the water off and put my clothes back on over wet skin; eyes shut tight against the engulfing mirror. Back in my room, sitting on my bed, is my dear friend Tanya, and in her arms is Ruby. I lose my breath.

'Ruby,' I whisper. She smiles. Perfection. Her eyes are so clear, and blue – the blue of the sky first thing in the morning. If I could paint her, I would paint her skin with marble dust and sun-thickened linseed oil and beeswax. I would paint her superbly round head and her hands, her nose, her feet, her baby buttocks. When she smiles her three-tooth-smile, something happens to my insides. A warmth. A warmth that slips down from my brain and slides along my spinal cord and then spreads out through my heart to my fingertips and toes. I gather her up into the centre of me, I let her grasp my breast, pull my nose and I screw up my face and she laughs. I cradle her head; her fairy-fine hair and her eyes and her skin – oh all of her – merus, angelus.

We drive into the city for coffee. The air is salty and cool.

death is gathering

He leans in and leers but I have Ruby in my arms. Suddenly I can smell it, the beautiful slightly bitter smell of strong black coffee and there's a rush of saliva in my mouth and the air is salty and cool and I have Ruby in my arms and whoosh, my heart is here, my lungs, I am present.

Damien and I talk about the business of getting better. We talk about the importance of space and time and the importance of being heard.

'There's no such thing as justice,' I say, sadly. 'Those folk who are the sickest, who are terribly, awfully completely lost in the serpent arms of psychiatric illness, who need the most space and time, we're herded in and out of the acute public units like cattle.'

'Very often we provide a place when no-one else will,' says Damien. 'And when no-one else can.'

'There is no such thing as justice,' I say to Aaron later in the therapy room.

'Yes. How are you sleeping?' he asks.

'Huh. If you were to turn us into a mathematical equation, each of us a straight line with a relationship to the x axis and the y axis, we'd probably intersect at infinity.'

'You do make things difficult,' he says.

'Shrinks,' I say to Zoë and Naava, as we sit drinking coffee in the hospital cafe. 'How can I be real, and open and honest and fragile when Aaron is so closed off he might as well be an automaton?'

'I agree,' Zoë says, sadly.

'It reminds me of the Sanskrit expression, Namaste: the spirit in me recognises and honours the spirit in you. The light within me honours the light within you. But when the spirit and the light are withheld so completely . . .'

'Finding the right psychiatrist is not the same as finding the right orthopaedic surgeon,' Naava says, staring into her coffee. Then she looks up and we hold eyes and grin at each other.

'I mean, the point of a therapeutic relationship is that it be therapeutic,' I say. 'It makes up about 30 percent of the whole healing thing.'

'30 per cent?'

'Yup. Certified evidence-based medicine.'

We sit for a while amid the hospital flotsam.

'You know what it's like, you want to feel kinda respected and listened to,' I say. 'There's nothing worse then being dismissed or ignored, even when you're really sick. I know pharmacotherapy is important and crisis care is important and education is important, but there's got to be more to it than that. Half the time I think Aaron is just trying to stay awake. Christ, I must be boring.'

Later in the day Sarah visits and brings a phalaenopsis orchid with four blazingly white flowers. Sarah and I have been firm friends since we were 12 years old. She's eight months pregnant with her second child. How stark the contrast between us. How good it is to see her. How it hurts.

Morning. Belinda, who has the room next to ours, is sitting in the courtyard drinking coffee and smoking.

'It's good to be thinking straight,' she says.

I sit down opposite. 'Hell yeah.'

'One day I was making a cup of coffee and I realised that if I poured the boiling water over my hands, they wouldn't burn, I mean I'd become sort of invincible, and I kept telling everyone because it was so amazing and no-one believed me and I got so bloody angry and so they stuffed me in HDU for four frigging weeks! Actually, I think I did need to be there cos I was off my head, I remember one of the nurses in HDU kept telling us stories about him being an astronaut in another life and I totally believed him! Oh my god, I was on so much frigging zyprexa, I put on six kilos in four weeks, how bad is that? I just kept on eating eating eating . . . and smoking cos there's nothing else to do in HD. D'you know, I quit for a year until this last episode and now I'm back on a pack a day.'

'It sucks,' I say. 'Going mad.'

'Fucking sucks,' Belinda says.

The Presence has slid out of my consciousness and divested Himself from my body. I accept that my brain conjured Him; I don't know why. Neurotransmitters have a part to play: dopamine, serotonin, noradrenaline, but there is a difference between what we conceptualise as the brain (purely organic) and what we conceptualise as the mind, and He definitely lived in my mind.

Damien asks if I will have a chat with some first year nursing students and I agree and we sit together in one of the therapy rooms.

'The thing with psychosis, with delusional thinking is . . .' I stop and sigh, trying to find the words. 'It's . . . well, when I'm sick I believe the delusional stuff to the same degree that you might know and believe the sky is above and the earth below. And if someone were to say to me that the delusional thinking is, in fact, delusional, well that's the same as if I assure you now that we walk on the sky. Of course you wouldn't believe me, and that's why it's sometimes so hard for people who are sick like this to accept treatment – to know that they even need treatment.'

The students are polite. They treat me like a bomb that may go off at any second.

'The other thing about psychosis and also severe depression is that they have a huge effect on how you relate to other people and how you see the world. It's a bit like being in a vacuum, or behind a wall of really thick glass . . . you lose any sense of connectedness. You're cast adrift from everyone and everything that matters. Some people never find a way back.'

After the students leave I shake hands with the nursing staff and pack up my books and music and a few clothes. Naava and I exchange phone numbers.

'Keep safe,' I say, hugging her gently.

'You too. See you on the outside.'

Damien isn't on shift, so I write him a letter to return with his books and my parents drive me home.

Home. Beautiful cats with their soft fur and warm bodies and candescent eyes. Books. Here I am in the same room as Toni Morrison and William Faulkner and Keri Hulme and T.S. Eliot – minds and minds and minds. I run my hands over the tops and sides of the books, feel their spines, salivate. My parents have stacked the freezer with food and cleaned the flat and washed my clothes and I'm consequently torn between gratitude and shame.

It is a further week of insensibility before I heave up the courage to ring my manager to arrange a return to work. Again the flooding gratitude that this workplace is willing to take me back at all after six weeks leave. The shame. In the intervening fortnight, I manage two things: driving from home to the cinema to see a children's film with my father, and walking to a local cafe for coffee with Melyse, after which on both occasions, I fall fast into a kind of catatonia deeper than the sea.

Naava comes to stay for a couple of weeks after her discharge from the inpatient unit. We sit together on the couch, smoking sweet, apple-flavoured tobacco through her water pipe.

'You okay?' she asks softly.

'Yeah.' I pause. Summon something like courage. All the years of building layer upon layer of internal fortification make it hard to admit I need someone. 'Glad I'm not alone,' I say.

'Yeah?' The ends of her mouth twitch.

'You okay?' I ask.

She nods, eyes all tears.

We don't go out much or sleep much or say much but we listen together to Dave Matthews and Tim Reynolds and we cook together and check that the other is taking her right medication. On bad nights one will wrap the other in (1) an enormous faux-fur blanket and (2) both arms. We shore each other up like two elderly, shallow-rooted trees, side-by-side in a high wind.

With Zoë, we spend long evenings discussing Life, and whether anyone has ever really had any idea about the whole soggy point of it. We eat smoked ocean trout and stuffed vine leaves and pita bread and olives. We ruminate about meaning and relationships and loneliness and illness. In the absence of partners of our own, we form what we call an 'emotional family,' meaning we'll be here for each other no matter what.

25

At the end of my first month back at work, there's a letter from Aaron's rooms in the mailbox. It's soggy where rain has seeped through cracks in the brick. I slide a finger under the edge of the envelope while driving to the library. It's a typed letter. A long typed letter. I pull over on the side of the road, under a streetlight. And then I take a long breath in . . . and forget to breathe out.

I've been dumped by my psychiatrist. This is not something I'd considered – Duty of Care and the Hippocratic Oath and all that. He says, in part, that I have poor insight and symptoms of psychosis. He says I'm not always compliant with his recommended treatment and I'm not always honest. His professional opinion is that my prognosis is of serious concern. He suggests I either re-connect with the Community Clinic or find another clinician. He wishes me well for the future.

I fold the letter in half and sharpen the crease and then I fold it in half again and sharpen the crease and then I fold it in half again and sharpen the crease. Once home from the library I put the fat little square of paper in the rubbish bin.

So my confusion about Psychiatry as a discipline solidifies. It was a vague mistrust in the beginning, a nebulous sense that something about the nature of the practice wasn't right.

As a medical student on psych rotations, the psychiatrists who taught us showed a modicum of respect and interest in the patients while in front of the patients (as professionalism dictates) but once we were closeted in an office, they'd discuss various symptoms as though they were disconnected from ever belonging to a human being. Sometimes they'd disbelieve a patient we'd interviewed some-what condescendingly, or flat-out dismiss another patient's suffering. One psychiatrist said, as I was shadowing him on a public unit, 'This place is a zoo. Get into private practice as soon as you can if you do psychiatry.'

The debilitating side effects of high dose antipsychotics like men-tal clouding, lethargy and sedation were glossed over. One feels (every hour of every day) the slow drowsiness of having drunk a lot of alco-hol without any of the associated pleasure or relaxation or emotional warmth. I wondered (then and now) if it would make a difference if these doctors themselves just once tried a low dose of the drugs they were prescribing.

Eight months away from becoming doctors ourselves, we'd had almost no teaching about the ways mental illness cause disruption to the lives of family and friends as well as to that of the sufferer, and we had little insight into the often life-long associated disability. No one ever said, 'Ethan over there was a highly functioning young man with a job and a lover and dreams and ambition and hope for the future. He was brought into hospital in the back of a Police van. Can you imagine the grief and confusion that must come with a diagnosis of manic-depression?'

There is always a power imbalance between a patient and physi-cian, but I've witnessed it more acutely in psychiatry than in almost any other branch of medicine. 'Them And Us.' And never the twain shall meet.

But Winsome chooses not to give up on me.

'I fully understand that all is not well and that you have been in a terrible space. It is good that you are still alive,' she says at our first session since my discharge from the inpatient unit.

'Winsome,' I say. 'I'm sorry.'

'Please do not apologise. You are in no way to blame.'

I look up from the floor fast, right into her eyes. My eyes. Hers. Oh, relief. I smile for the first time in weeks. 'I was difficult and I feel bad about that. But thank you. I seem to have regained my rational mind.'

'Wonderful,' she says. 'For better or worse, the last eight weeks are murky and confused – until I woke up on Sunday and felt myself.'

Winsome smiles. 'What a relief for you.'

'I think . . . I hope . . . the blackness and the paranoia is not all of who I am.'

'I agree.'

'Coming here this morning I was scared you might have had enough.'

'Of?'

'This. Me. Us.'

Winsome waits, not staring at me, but just with her presence, creating space (in which to be honest).

'Um, because this means a lot. This. Us. I pay you, it's professional and so on, I know that. Still.'

'And we'll work together till you get there Kate. You will get there.'

I'm running on a beach, flat, hot, beautiful sand, water, waves, flying.

For a second.

But it's good.

'Do you think there is such a thing as a psychiatrist who sees the whole person – I mean really sees the whole person?' I ask.

'I don't know,' says Winsome.

'Damn it Winsome, all the facets of the human condition exist in a person with mental illness. Right?'

'Right.'

'Desire, love . . . search for meaning. Connection. Pain.'

'Yes. Absolutely.'

'D'you know, the literal translation of psychiatry is healing of the soul.'

We sit quietly with this.

Winsome moves her consulting room to a comfortable cream Edwardian with tall roses in the front garden. The chairs are deep and soft. The courtyard has cumquat trees in pots around its edges. The cumquats are the glowing orange of just-blown-on-coals.

'We all have a presentable face – a self that is socially acceptable and professionally acceptable,' Winsome says. 'Yes?'

'Yes.'

'Here we are exploring the much deeper stuff. All the layers underneath.'

'Yes.'

'And some of your layers have been hidden for a long time, and there is a lot of pain.'

I nod.

no kill her

'Can you tell me more about the pain?'

do it do it hands throat THROAT

There appear to be clouds in the room.

'It's awfully crowded . . .' I tap my head with my index finger. Tap. Tap. Then I hunch up. There are clouds in the room.

'Crowded,' Winsome says.

'Foreverandeverandever,' I whisper to the rug. My boots are purple.

'Pardon?'

'Clouds.'

Winsome's eyes are the only light. 'Tell me what is going on . . . in your mind . . . right now.'

Silence-and-clouds and

is-there-an-I and

are-they-going-to-let-me-live.

'Do you think everyone has . . .?'

'Has . . .?' says Winsome. Her voice is measured, soft.

'Other . . . I know there's the self . . .'

'Yes.'

'Here,' I tap my head. Tap. Tap. 'There's a sort-of-self, a theoretical self, at least I think so, because I'm saying I . . .'

I stare at my boots. My boots are purple. Winsome thinks there are two of us in this room, but she is wrong.

kill her

Time diffracts.

'Sometimes the thing called self disappears completely. There's an awful lot of black. Black bile, black dog, Black Death, and . . . I'm kind of governed.

Actually, I'm kind of suffocated.'

Hunched up. The rug is Turkish. My voice is over the other side of the room. The people in my head are going to kill her for this line of questioning, but Winsome is relaxed; still – in her chair, her neat feet quiet on the floor. She isn't bothered by the clouds.

'Kate,' she says. 'You are safe here.' She pauses. 'You are safe enough to tell the truth.' She pauses. 'Who is suffocating you?'

'There's um, there's quite a lot of them,' I say.

Now the shaking. Thighs, knees. Nipples tight shut.

'They live . . .'

Winsome's expression hasn't changed. She doesn't look like she's trying not to laugh. I open up my hands. There are little sweat-rivers in the palmar creases.

'They live . . .' I tap my head with my index finger. Tap. Tap. 'Here.'

The room has shrunk; the walls folding into a cylinder, pressing. Low cloud like fog . . . and where is the light? Winsome's eyes keep me from dying.

'Years and years and years and years and years and years and years. Jesus.'

do it do it hands throat THROAT

'Sometimes they rage,' I whisper. 'Sometimes it's do this, do this and then they laugh.'

And then my breath runs out.

Gag.

shhhh

'Shhhh,' I whisper. Frozen. I have given them up – a betrayal, and they are like Medusa: snaky-headed, potent gazed. Perseus severed Medusa's head from her body and not even that curtailed her power. Poisonous vipers grew from the spilt drops of her blood.

you bitch

this is the end

They are in unison. They are around my throat and my life is in my throat and air isn't moving anymore and evidently this is the end.

Winsome waits until my breathing rights itself. After a long time I look up and nod and smile and wipe the sweat from around my eyes and lips.

'Jesus,' I say in my ordinary voice. 'The clouds have gone.' I move forward in the seat to stand up but my knees won't straighten.

'Take your time,' Winsome says.

'Sorry,' I say, flushing and suddenly cold. I look up again. The room is cream and softly lit and I'm still alive. I've told someone about . . . and I'm fucking well still alive.

All night I sit in bed with cats asleep around me and think. Meaning. Illness. Ordinary life. The beauty of ordinary life and the enormousness of *their* power, *their* truth, *their* meaning. The cats stretch and sigh, air fluffing through their noses. Their eyelids flutter as they dream. On my bedroom wall is Marc Chagall's painting, *Three Candles*: a twilight world of rapt figures in which the gold candles throw yellow through blue and lovers embrace the sky in a dreamy elegance; their hands touch among fruiting lilacs. Orange angels populate the boughs with fully fleshed bodies attached to wings ethereal as cotton flowers. It is enough.

In the morning I walk to the train station with the sun low in the eastern sky. The air feels new in my mouth and lungs. The people in my head are hissing as usual and I can feel the heat of their eyes but I can also hear Winsome's voice, low and soft, 'You are safe'. So I get on the train, stand in the corner of the carriage, headphones on, books clutched, and I get off at the right station and go to work. And all through the day and into the evening when I walk from work into the city, I wonder . . . at the possibility . . . that *their* truth may not be the truth.

I've believed them, all of them, since I was sixteen – fifteen years of bitter acumen, sarcasm, bile and vomit, fifteen years of their ability to halve and quarter me. I am naked before them and whenever they see my body their laughter is high and mirthless. They have always outwitted me.

And now. Given that I'm standing here on the steps of Flinders Street Station, oddly enough alive . . .

Oddly enough alive.

The dusk air carries with it the colours of the sunset – carmine red and cadmium scarlet and magenta – smooth as honey on my skin. I sit on the steps until the almostblack sky is above and all around. There are no stars.

A week later Winsome draws a picture of my brain.

'We know you have a presenting self – let's put that towards the front. Then there's the . . . cacophony, made up of the voices and their judgements and criticisms and bullying. And in between is a sliver of real self.'

'Real self? Huh.'

'Yes indeed. And one of our goals here is to manage the cacophony and to find some space in which the real self can grow.'

Then Winsome says, 'Who are you, Kate? What makes up your real self?'

I think about this for a while. 'Most of the time, about twenty percent of me is alive in the external world and the rest flails about . . . mired, stammering . . . in the internal world.'

'That must be very tiring,' says Winsome.

'Yes.'

eeeeeeee shhhh die do it doit THROAT

I close my eyes. Put my hands around my throat.

'Take your hands away from your throat, Kate,' says Winsome. 'Tell me what's happening.'

Her voice is safe.

I sit on my hands to keep them under control.

I take a breath.

Then I say, very quietly, 'There were only three of them to begin with – BANG – when I was sixteen. I don't know where they came from. At first I kept looking around to see if anyone else heard them shouting, but no one ever did. And then I assumed everyone had, you know, *other* . . . but that it was something private, like vaginitis, so I never said anything and I practiced a pleasant face. No matter what they said . . . no matter what they said, I trained myself not to react. Now when they order me to do things, I do it with a smile.'

Winsome doesn't look aghast and nor is she laughing. 'Thank you for sharing this with me,' she says. 'How did you train yourself not to react?'

'All I could think of at the time was spies – this group of people who successfully lead double lives. I read everything I could about techniques of espionage and counterintelligence, all the biographies, memoirs and straight non-fiction, mostly from the Cold War, and then I put what I learned into practice at home and school.'

'What sort of things?'

'It's embarrassing, Winsome.'

She waits.

'Feeling one thing, physically and emotionally, and at the same time expressing the opposite. I practised sticking a sewing needle in my arm while chatting to friends on the phone or giggling, that kind of thing.'

'Why?'

'So when the people in my head shouted . . . stuff . . . no-one else would ever know.'

Winsome shakes her head. 'These voices may be a part of you, but they are not all of you.' She pauses. 'And they are telling you lies.' She pauses. 'Let's think about how we're going to manage them.'

eeeeeeeee shhhhdie

I nod, lips tight shut, not-breathing. The smallest core of hope has lodged itself like a light, somewhere near my heart.

The first thing we do is to devise a way of surviving the supermarket: Sennheiser noise-cancelling headphones. With music up loud I can't hear the people in my head as clearly and by focussing on melody and lyrics, I'm somewhat disconnected from the mountains of competing colour on the shelves. We try other potential filters like breathing exercises and stillness meditation but they are less successful.

Because evenings are most difficult, Winsome suggests structuring the time with normal activities like gardening or cooking, and reducing stimuli – be it aural, visual, kinaesthetic or emotional. We explore ways to 'wind down' that don't involve alcohol or other drugs.

The answer for me is cello. The violoncello is a member of the violin family, bigger than a viola, smaller than a double bass. There is something about the cello sound – its full, burnished tone, its richness, its ability to lament. Between the instrument and the musical score and the musician, everything is communicated without a need for words.

There is also a physicality to playing an instrument that I love – the sheen of the wood, the conifer-smell of rosin, the strings under my fingers, the bow on the strings. And the repetition of practice is meditative in a way traditional meditation is not, because my attention is drawn out of me and focused wholly on hand position and vibrato and sliding shifts and bow change and intonation.

Winsome and I have been working together for two years now, and for the next ten months we work particularly hard. I see her once a week. She stresses the importance of addressing both halves of my divided brain – the normal and the abnormal.

'Our aim,' she says, 'is balance and eventual wholeness.'

She is patient and consistent. It takes another two months before I can turn up to an appointment without an enormous bag of books and six layers of clothes. One evening we spend a whole session – close to ninety minutes – writing a 'normal' grocery list.

'What is normal to eat for breakfast, Kate?'

I frown. 'Coffee.'

'By itself, no.'

I glare. 'Air.'

Winsome glares right back. 'Do not play games with me. It is a waste of your time, and mine.'

The fast flush. The sudden rush of red.

'We are working together,' she says gently. 'I can see that that in itself is challenging for you – the process of trust.'

She's right.

'I like oatmeal,' I say, my voice pathetic and low.

'Could you have oatmeal and a piece of fruit?'

I think. 'Okay. Yes.'

We talk about going to the supermarket to buy oatmeal and fruit.

We spent weeks discussing how to structure a normal day. If I'm up till 3 a.m. writing poetry, Winsome says, 'Kate, this isn't normal. Did you concentrate properly at work?'

No.

If I leap out of bed and walk into the city because I suddenly have to buy some poetry, Winsome says, 'Risky behaviour. Please don't wander around the city at night on your own. It isn't safe.'

She never lets anything go till we work it through.

'It's normal to get a haircut at a hairdresser,' she says. 'And it's fun. It's normal to find a bra that fits properly. It's normal to wear clothes of an appropriate size – clothes that are comfortable for the climate and season.'

And she never lets anything go.

Once I manage a reasonable daily routine, we shift focus in therapy to the idea of mind-body-spirit in equilibrium. I am afraid of the body. The concepts of 'nourishment' and 'pleasure' for the body are incomprehensible.

'Nourishment might be cooking a simple, healthy meal or going for a walk.' Winsome says. 'Pleasure might be buying and wearing silky lingerie.'

I swallow awkwardly.

She waits for my brain to catch up. 'Or you could sink into a warm, perfumed bath.'

Now I've forgotten how to swallow.

'You could have sex.'

'Outré.'

'C'est normale.'

She waits.

After a while I breathe out properly. We both half-smile. Eyes and minds stretching and meeting.

26

Some weekends I drive out of the city. Under a tree is the best place in the world to think, preferably where there are lots of trees – trees and silence and sky. I sit cross-legged under a manna gum just off a walking track in the middle of the Mornington Peninsula National Park and wonder about meaning and illness and the beauty of ordinary life. Can I have an ordinary life? What about the idea of a future?

The surrounding eucalypts, banksias and xanthorrhoea grasstrees remind me of Gondwana. Rhoea is Greek for flow. As well as having sap that flows down the trunk, the leaves of the grasstree look like a green waterfall, and the parts of the National Park where the grasstrees grow thick appear to be spouting and streaming, and within some, a black flower spike two metres tall, broader than my arm, is heading straight for the centre of the sky. Grasstrees have been around for 200 million years. Such resilience.

I wonder whether meaning is connected to pleasure. And then I wonder if addiction is pleasure without meaning. Addiction is certainly connected to illness. And illness is connected to future. The trees soak into my guts and still the shouting in my head. I make a decision: I will get off the benzos.

The brain is a delicate thing, not much given to sudden changes in its environment. If it adapts over time to a constant supply of benzodiazepine, then that supply becomes as necessary for daily functioning as glucose and water. I wake to the sound of music emanating from next door – Yo La Tengo. The bass runs through me. I will get off the benzos. Quietly, with the minimum of fuss, my own little experiment with the forces of addiction.

There is a website that counsels addicts on methods of dose reduction and withdrawal. I sign up as a new member and read that it can take a year or more to fully withdraw, a few milligrams of diazepam at a time. It is an incremental process because benzodiazepines directly or indirectly influence almost every aspect of brain function. They increase the activity of a neurotransmitter called GABA which is the brain's natural tranquiliser. Over time, an addict's brain like mine gets used to this tranquiliser effect, and begins to crave more and more of it just to feel normal.

I gather up the blister packs of lorazepam and alprazolam and the bottle of clonazepam and empty them into the toilet bowl where they disperse blue and yellow and white lines of powder that rise toward the surface of the water. I flush and walk away.

It is autumn. Next-door's crepe myrtle has caught fire. The air has a heavy warmth during the day and a sweet crispness at night. Streetlights come on earlier; people bend slightly into the wind. The first 24 hours without benzos passes. I go to work, I come home, I don't sleep. My jaw is so heavy I find it difficult to eat. Then I find it difficult to speak. Muscles in my neck and upper back spasm, my legs jerk suddenly in the night and now that it is morning, every hair on the pillow is sending an individual signal to the sensory cortex of my brain. I'm not quite sure how to get out of bed. The wind through the trees is a thousand ghosts, whispering, intent. I try opening and closing my eyes one at a time but my eyelashes get caught under my lower eyelid and all I can see is the long black of spiders' legs.

On the third day I sit cross-legged just beneath the ceiling in the corner of the room and watch my body below. I watch the body interact with other people, I watch it lie on the bed – frumpish, round-shouldered and fat. Speech becomes an exercise in chance, walking an exercise in the fragility of balance. The opening of the train carriage door, on my way to work, is as miraculous as the opening of Tutankhamun's tomb – letting in of the light. It takes half an hour longer than ever before to walk from the station because the ground is alternately rising up and sinking as though I am at sea. Within the rises and falls I negotiate putting one foot in front of the other. Sometimes I fail and find myself on outstretched hands and knees, the tips of my fingers curled into the ground to prevent myself from falling off the ends of the world.

Once at my desk I turn on the computer. The icons on my desktop are little dobs of fuzzy colour; emails are dark grey clouds on a white background. My handwriting is unrecognisable.

'You are very quiet,' people from work say. I smile and try to nod without my head falling off. 'Busy,' I say. 'Reports.' Later, I say to my dear friend and colleague, Deborah, 'I'm feeling a bit weird – I think I'll sit in the library for a while. Page me if anything comes up?' she nods. 'Sorry,' I say.

'It's okay,' she says.

I sit in the library with closed eyes – whenever I open them, the books are moving around on their shelves. I am subject to tics, odd sensations, confusion. I can't tell the time of day. Light enters my eye and lingers there, shivering slightly. The sky is too bright. If I rub my hands together I cannot quite feel where one begins and the other ends.

At night the sea enters me, my legs and arms ripple at random, the sides of the room merge with the roof and settle themselves there before sliding back to the floor. I listen to the radio and grasp at the voices – they have an animate form. The radio sound stretches and sways, it looms overhead and then narrows into the hush of a conch shell. Time is capricious. The people in my head flicker and bicker. They take up an enormous amount of space. Sometimes I hear them whispering just behind my right ear. I turn suddenly but they turn with me and remain out of reach.

Naava and I have tickets for a gig at the Corner Hotel in Richmond. I'm interested to see how my body will respond to music. Naava helps me out of the car and up the three steps like I'm ninety years old and in need of a walking frame. A string of clear light globes loops across the roof of the stage. In the dark as the lights flash on-off-on the filaments, frail metal, flower like gold. I merge into the people around me as waves into the sea; they rock and sway inside me. My head splits open to receive the music – its rawness is sandpaper approaching grey and white matter.

On the sixth day there is a soft sheen of fluid over my irises. The hairs on my arms and legs are erect; goose-pimpled. My heartbeat is insistent against my chest, the air palpable on my skin. On the eighth day I can swallow again and wrap my fingers around a glass of water and bring it smoothly to my lips. Water falls into my mouth like rain.

To manage phone calls at work, I listen politely and write down as much as I can in point form and I say, 'Thank you, I'll look into this and call you back in ten minutes,' and I hang up and pinch myself hard to release some adrenaline and then I read the words in my stuttering hand over and over until they make some sense.

On the tenth day I peel myself off the roof and begin to walk in straight lines, but it is another week before I can own my limbs and my breathing. Life without benzos lends the world a sharpness, it is acute angles and white light and voices that sound out a white intensity. It is like getting glasses for the first time, like seeing the delicacy of leaves on the trees and street signs sharp in the dusk. Benzo-free consciousness means acute concentration, thought that is fierce, that expands and sways, and memory that has a life of its own.

After four weeks I am normal enough to go out in the company of other, normal, people – my presence at work is too ghost-like to count. I'm sitting in a cafe not far from the sea. It has dark wooden panelling, dark wooden chairs, little light, which suits me perfectly. I take out my pile of books, given that reading is again possible. The shopkeeper brings coffee – strong and bitter and black. Then she turns around.

'Come on, you pigeons,' she says. 'Out.'

The pigeons continue further into the cafe, under the counter, around the counter, into the back room, their necks bobbing, beaks to the ground and then as they reach my feet, they tip their heads to the side – one orange-rimmed eye each on my eyes . . . my feet . . . my eyes.

'Hello you pigeons,' I say and I drop little pieces of cake under the table when the shopkeeper has her back turned – it is a rounded back, a soft curve from thoracic spine to neck. But the lines around her eyes and mouth are all old smiles. I drink the coffee, read, smile now and again to the shopkeeper and under the tablecloth the pigeons peck and swallow all of the cake.

'Do you believe in the concept of soul?' Winsome asks the following morning.

I haven't yet found a way to tell her about the benzos, so I think about this, I look at the roof. 'Yes.'

'Psychology is primarily a science, but there is also an element of art. Jung says it's a collision of nature and spirit.'

'I like that.'

'Thinking and feeling are equally important, as are perception and intuition and sensation and logic.'

I nod. 'I'm scared, Winsome.'

'What are you scared of?'

'It's mostly them, but I'm still scared you'll tell me quietly and professionally that I would be better off seeing someone else – like Aaron did.'

'I have never – and shall never suggest that you see another therapist. Though I do question your medication, because, whilst it holds you, more or less, it doesn't stop the agonising stuff that goes on in your head, does it?'

Right here, I realise she has just saved my life.

The sunlight is bright-eyed through the window.

'True,' I say.

'Tell me what's been happening . . . in your head.'

So I tell her. 'At night the hooded people come. They carry axes and long knives and I lie down on my stomach on the cold floor, naked, and they hack at my back, my skull – all that soft flesh. I know I'll die, but I do nothing. There is much blood, hot and red and black in the night. Sometimes the whole thing makes me smile. I really need my head drained, Winsome, I need a new brain. Iamasickfuck.'

Winsome listens, and then she says quietly, 'Your recovery is going to be a very slow and gentle process of trust and taking small steps. It is not always going down a cognitive, action-oriented path: it is much more about the emergence of the real self – the mind and body and spirit together.'

She stands up. 'I want you to keep telling those voices that they are shouting lies and that you won't put up with them anymore.'

When I walk outside there is a kaffir lime tree in a pot on the side of the road, shining. The rain, the smell of new rain, the way asphalt sings a little and the trees respond and right here, this kaffir lime tree on the side of the road is singing and shining and its double leaves, the newest ones, are midori green and there are drops of water on them reflecting my eye.

Benzodiazepines decrease time in REM sleep (dream sleep). Sleep without benzos is the people in my head and the dreams and me locked together in a cranial cavity fifty-seven centimetres in circumference. The frontal bone and the parietal bone, the temporal and occipital and sphenoid bones are articulated but not fused to allow moulding through the birth canal and later, growth of the brain, but they do not accommodate a way of escape from this violent phantasmagoria.

Is dreaming the closest a sane person can come to the experience of madness? Seventeenth-century physicians hypothesised that dreams and madness shared the same movement of vapours and animal spirits; the notion of waking was 'all that distinguished a madman from a man asleep.'

I moan and whine to Naava and Zoë about the dreams, about being awake more than half the night – sweating, tachycardic and breathless, and about reeling through the workday with blurred vision and a high b'zzzz in my ears.

'What about trying one of these?' Naava walks into my room holding a box of Pericyazine tablets. Pericyazine is an anti-psychotic, but some psychiatrists use a low dose for the symptoms of severe anxiety and insomnia because unlike benzodiazepines, it is not addictive and doesn't induce dependence. Tonight, I take a single 2.5 mg tablet and curl up in bed with fleece blankets and fat cats and the BBC World Service.

Two months on pericyazine, two tiny tablets at night, one at midday. The most extraordinary thing is happening – the people in my head are fainter, less insistent. There are whole hours when they disappear all together. And sleep. Oh blissful, beautiful sleep – for more than two hours in a row, for more than four hours in twenty-four. Mornings are new. I wake without the memory of the preceding night bitten into my brain, without the vague sense of horror. My pyjamas are dry and soft and they don't smell. Sun waves are reflecting from my neighbour's pool onto the bedroom wall and I've never seen anything so sleek or so tender.

Normal sleep is now thought to have an essential role in cognitive and emotional processing. Sleep deprivation decreases the metabolic activity of the brain, particularly in the prefrontal and parietal-associational areas. These are important for judgement, impulse control, attention and visual association. People with chronic sleep deprivation are usually unaware of the extent of their cognitive deficits.

'Winsome,' I say. 'I've started answering the telephone at home. And the television isn't leering at me at night when it's turned off. Who knows, next I might take the blankets off the mirrors, next I might even touch someone.'

'Wonderful,' she says. 'When are you going to see your doctor to discuss how to take this drug properly?'

'Ah . . .'

'What is the appropriate dose? How often should you take it?'

'I've done the research, I've read MIMS and the journals and the professional websites.'

'You must talk to an objective clinician. You of all people know the dangers of self-medication. And medication is not my area of expertise. Please make an appointment with Jenny this week.'

Winsome is a qualified counselling psychologist. This means she works with people experiencing problems in relationships, within family units and in times of great stress like bereavement and divorce. She provides psychotherapy for people with depression and anxiety but medication for serious mental illness is the domain of general medical practitioners like Jenny and psychiatrists.

Jenny listens while I explain how the slowly increasing dose of Pericyazine has had a linear, inverse relationship to the shouting in my head. We discuss side effects and agree on an appropriate dose.

'This is terrific,' she says, writing me a prescription. 'Keep going with it.'

For several months, I sleep twelve to fourteen hours straight. I'm obsessed with the concept of a regular, easy period of night-unconsciousness. I'm not sure, but I think my brain might be healing itself.

During the day, the process of thinking is untainted, uninfected; rather it is sequential and fluid. I have a capacity for learning new things; I'm interested in things. The fog . . . the turgid white fog has gone. I'm aware of my body – chest wall when I breathe, pectorals, biceps, finger bones. I'm also aware of people in the street, the smell of the air and the feel of the sun. There is room in my head, depths and hollows. I echo. Thinking takes up a different time and space so that it is as easy to get lost in it as within a deep cave; the dark vanishing somewhere overhead.

A friend from university and I go out for coffee and his voice is clear, in both annunciation and meaning. All of me is listening to him, absorbing him, all of me is right here in this cafe where his hair is reflecting the sun like water.

'It's bizarre,' I say. 'I can hear every word you say. I mean, I'm sure I always could, there's nothing wrong with my hearing, but I used to process every second or third word, or sometimes I'd only catch the very end of a sentence, because there'd be blah blah blah at the same time, and so I'd nod and smile and try to look like I understood and, oh God, just hope that the other person didn't notice.'

He sighs and shakes his head. 'Bloody hell.'

'Yeah. But I think I now understand what Thich Nhat Hanh means by being in the present moment.'

'My brother met Hanh once, at his sangha in France.'

'Really? I'd probably swoon on the spot. And then die of embarrassment.'

We laugh.

The palm trees along Jacka Parade are ruffling in the wind. 'I know it's not a cure,' I say quietly. 'I mean, I'm still dysfunctional. Just not, you know . . . *mad* and dysfunctional.'

Pericyazine 2.5 mg and 10 mg tablets. Pale yellow and white. 25 tablets in each blister pack. Four blister packs in every box. One hundred Pills For Sanity at $14.45 or $3.95 concession.

The dreadful urge to mutilate my body . . . vanishes that way thirst does after receiving water or a burning itch is soothed. The scars turn from red, raised and angry to finer white, and like lines or paths, they tell their own stories. Sensation to the skin isn't returning however, and hair grows only between patches of injury.

'I haven't existed properly, in this body,' I say to Winsome. 'Not for a long time.'

She nods.

'Feeling,' I touch my fingertips together. 'Flesh. A beginning. Is it? Does it?'

'What?'

'Bring connectedness. Between me, as in my mind, and the world.'

'Your body? Yes.'

'Hah. It's taken me awhile. What's this, about age two in the realm of developmental psychology?'

Winsome smiles. 'Two or three.'

'It was okay once. And then I lost it.'

'I suspect you are right.'

'So it occurs to me that my once carefully constructed reality is, in fact, false – I mean, to the point of being delusional.'

'Yes,' she says.

'So maybe I do have a mental illness.

Fuck that hurts.

Winsome sits quietly. Then she says, 'This is a breakthrough for you.'

I wave my hands – comme ci comme ça. 'I'm still uneasy. About taking a drug that alters my brain . . . I mean, alters the way I think, what I think, how I respond to the world. It's a weird concept.' I scrunch up my eyes, rub my forehead hard. 'And Rose and Henry have left so I'm a bit bereft.'

'Rose and Henry?'

'Oh, you know, my companions of a sort. They loved each other. In here,' I tap the side of my head with my index finger.

There's an article in the paper today about volunteer-fostering very new kittens and sick or abused cats from a local animal shelter. I apply, go for an interview, pass a police check, attend a training session with other feline-centric people. My first foster cats are a pair of young adult brothers, all white and terrified of everything, especially me. They sit rod-still in their carry-box, eyes black pupil with the thinnest yellow rim. I set up their food and water and litter in the bathroom and line the bath with thick, soft blankets, tip the carry-box onto its side and ease them out. They're thin and shivering. They hiss and stick their claws into the back of my hands. They bite.

'It's okay, young ones. It's okay now.'

I leave them for the evening but every night after work, I sit in the other end of the bath with a book and a glass of wine. We sit for hours, none of us moving, just checking each other out. Their stiff crouches ease. One cat yawns. One white paw stretches in my direction. Two.

I smile.

Then the phone rings; the moth-soft paws retract. I go out to answer the phone and when I get back, both cats are over my side of the bath.

'Boys, what are you doing?'

Two white heads, wet whiskers. Between them they've lapped up half a glass of white wine. The cats settle back in their corner.

'No more wine. Is that clear?'

They stare. Silent. Candle-flame eyes.

27

There is so much about the functioning of the brain that we still don't understand. This is true for neurological function and psychological function and for the delicate connections between the two.

A study of 3300 UK adults born in 1946 who had a psychiatric examination at age 36 were then followed up until the age of 60. The results, published in 2011, showed that individuals diagnosed with a psychiatric disorder had an 84 per cent higher chance of dying before the age of 60 than those without. The increase was not accounted for by suicide, physical health or socio-economic factors. 'It is remarkable,' the authors wrote, that an interview on mood and thinking administered as a one off test at 36 years of age 'appears to impact on mortality more than two decades later.' Why? The reasons remain unclear.

But Mental Health is not sexy. Pharmaceutical companies fund very little research in the field of mental health in comparison with their investments in cancer, kids and cardiovascular disease.

Professor of Psychiatry at Monash University, Jayashri Kulkarni says, 'there is one big piece of the jigsaw puzzle that still seems to be missing in Australia's commitment to mental health: investment in clinical mental health research. Despite the raw facts – mental illness is the third-highest cause of disability and premature death in Australia and one in four of us will experience mental illness in our lifetime – only 3.5 per cent of Australia's total medical research budget is spent on research into depression and psychosis.'

There's a small, relatively new centre of psychiatry research in Melbourne and I ring to see if I'm eligible to participate in one of their clinical trials. Over the next 18 months I take part in three studies. One is an observational exploration of treatments and outcomes in people with a history of bipolar or schizoaffective disorder.

Baseline results show that half of the 240 participants smoke daily, less than half are in a stable relationship, over a third are unemployed and two thirds contemplated suicide in the month prior to entering the study. Like me, there is an average seven-year gap between first onset of symptoms and first medical treatment. That's seven years of confusion and problematic mood swings and periodic terror.

Hopefully the field of neuropsychiatry will continue to expand with advances in imaging of the structure and function of the brain. In time, it may be possible to identify genes or critical DNA variants, patterns of electrical activity, neurotransmitter levels or neuroanatomical abnormalities that confer susceptibility to illnesses such as schizophrenia and bipolar disorder.

Such tests could immediately identify individuals at risk and be a useful adjunct to diagnosis. For example it is now clear, 'that dopamine dysfunction is the final common pathway to developing psychotic symptoms,' says Professor Sir Robin Murray, from the Institute of Psychiatry at King's College London. Dopamine is one of the brain's neurotransmitters that effects communication between neurones (brain cells).

With regard to schizophrenia, Professor Murray says 'Excessive dopamine leads to salience being attached to ideas and objects that are, in fact, unimportant. The number of red cars that you passed on the way to work, or the fact that two people coughed at the same time, takes on new meanings.'

One day we may have very specific, molecularly targeted treatments for mental illness similar to those already in use for cancer. Compliance with current medication regimes is a real problem because of intolerable side effects. Research into psychosocial interventions including supportive care and psychotherapy remains equally valuable.

'The important thing,' says Professor Kulkarni 'is to find what works.'

Zoë is terribly sick. Like Naava and myself, she has battled more than one episode of severe depression before adulthood.

'It sits in the back of my mind all the time, you know?' she says.

Saturday nights the three of us are lounging on couches at my place or hers for food and wine and honesty.

'No matter where I am or what I'm doing, it's always there. It's in my dreams.'

We know.

The thoughts that give no peace. And the ache. The grief that is not really grief. The damn endless, endless misery.

Suicide.

'Are you getting any sleep?' Naava asks.

'Three or four hours.'

'Shit.' We say it together.

'But I didn't actually get out of bed till four this afternoon,' Zoë says. 'And I'm more exhausted in the mornings than I am in the evenings.'

She's subsisting on chocolate and nicotine, self-medication of sorts. She has a wonderful psychologist and a supportive doctor, but severe depression locks the mind in a scold's bridle. It's an unreachable despair.

One evening Zoë rings from an Emergency Department.

'I um . . . I cut myself,' she says. 'I'll be home soon. Can you come over?'

I do and we hug in the hallway and I wish I could transmit more than physical warmth.

'What's happening, honey?' I ask.

We sit close together on her couch. She doesn't answer for a long time.

She says, 'I hate feeling like absolute shit every single fucking day. It's HELL.'

Keep quiet and calm. Quiet and calm. Don't cry. 'Oh Jesus,' I say softly. 'I'm so sorry.'

Quiet and calm. Don't cry.

'I can't keep going like this,' she says.

Tears run down my face over my chin and drip onto my t-shirt.

'Please,' I say. 'We can get through this.'

She shakes her head.

'I love you,' I say.

'I'm sorry.'

We both cry harder.

'He was an arsehole,' she says after a while, eyes on the floor.

'Who?'

'He treated me – not like an animal – more like a slab of meat.'

'Who did?'

'The emergency doctor.'

'What happened?'

'First I waited for three hours. I know I didn't have a life-threatening emergency, I know that, but it was bloody hard to sit there with all these people and not completely freak out.'

'Three hours.'

'Yep. Then they put me in the procedure room and just left me,

204

with boxes of scalpels and needles and whatever else and they knew I was there because of self-harm.'

'You're fucking kidding.'

'Then the doctor came in.'

Zoë stares at the floor. Not blinking, not crying anymore. I fold my hands to keep them still and wait.

'He hardly said a word to me,' she says. 'He didn't even wait for the local anaesthetic to kick in, he just started suturing and when I said, excuse me, it's really hurting, he mumbled something like, well it must have hurt to do it in the first place. Like he was punishing me.'

I look at her wounds. Deep red cries. Deep red pain. The stitches are uneven – some tight, some loose – and they're too far apart. It's a shoddy job. I try adding some steri-strips so the wounds won't re-open before her own doctor can review them tomorrow. There's an engineer's vice in the centre of my chest and it's crushing my heart on both sides.

'How're you doing?' I ask her later.

'Scared shitless. How're you doing?'

'Scared shitless.'

The following week, Zoë's doctor goes on holiday and Zoë again requires stitches for deep cuts to her legs and belly. She is drifting further away from us, closing down, her voice is low and flat, her face, her eyes . . . her eyes were like that first touch of sunlight through clear, deep water. Now they are grey.

When the thoughts of suicide are absolute and unshakeable, she makes an appointment to see her doctor's covering clinician. He refuses to admit her to the clinic where she's been an inpatient before, where she has some connection with the staff and the place itself. In his learned opinion, the hospital environment is counterproductive for some people. After reviewing Zoë once, for fifteen minutes, he decides she is one of those people.

If I were in any way inclined to violence . . .

We try to make an appointment to see my GP, Jenny, who is also on holiday. Her covering clinician listens carefully and rings the intake co-ordinators of all the private psychiatric hospitals in Melbourne. There are no beds available. We sit in the waiting room while she sees other patients. Then we go back in and she tries the public units. There are no beds available.

'What are we going to do?' I ask.

'I'm so sorry,' she says. 'Come back and see me tomorrow and we'll try again.'

The three of us hunch up on the couch at my place with comfort food and vodka. We're not hungry. Naava and I wait till Zoë has taken her medication – antidepressants and a sleeping tablet. When she's drowsy, Naava and I take our own medication and we all get into my bed. The cats curl up with us.

At 5 a.m. there's just a hint of light through the window and I can see Zoë's chest rising and falling as she breathes. She's breathing too slowly.

"Zoë, are you okay?' I shake her gently. Naava is awake now.

'Is she okay?' she asks.

'No.'

I ring triple zero. 'My friend has taken an overdose sometime in the night, I think. She's breathing, but she's unconscious.'

While we wait for the ambulance, the operator says, 'Count out her pulse for me.'

'One, two, three . . .'

'Now count out her breaths.'

'One . . . two . . .'

The paramedics arrive and they insert an oro-pharyngeal tube to help with her breathing and give her some high flow oxygen and I sit next to the driver and we travel with lights and sirens to the hospital. Once there, Naava and I are ushered into 'the relatives room.' I know this room – it's where they put people whose loved ones are either critically ill or already dead. Soft lighting, a telephone, a box of tissues. Naava and I don't speak. Everything is blurry. One of the emergency physicians comes in.

'She's going to be okay,' he says.

I feel like a block of ice receiving the sun.

'We've had to intubate her so she'll be in intensive care for a few days.'

I ring Zoë's family, who are interstate but will get on a plane immediately. At home I sit on the front steps. It is raining. Light is lavishing sheen onto a puddle of water at my feet. Water falling several millilitres at a time into water. Water responding with wavelets, rings, circles that are, in spite of everything, radiating and concentric and perfect. Then I go inside and lie down and howl.

When we visit the next day, Zoë is awake. I reach for both her hands, holding them in mine, so tight. Not letting go. We sit here, not moving. The cubicle curtains shift as people walk past. Someone's mobile rings out hip-hop. My left hand cramps, Zoë's hands, inside mine, are turning dark red-blue. We sit here, not moving. Then she looks at me and at my eyes that are saying the same thing as my hands and if I could only transplant into her – so that she believed it – the preciousness of her life.

Why does it so often take a serious act of harm to self or others before someone is deemed sick enough to be admitted to hospital?

'I don't understand,' I say to Zoë's parents. They are looking shattered. Zoë spends the next eight weeks in the clinic from which she was previously refused admission. On discharge she's somewhat stable, but it's many months for her, I think, before the idea of death is unreservedly supplanted by the idea of living.

The Australian Institute for Patient and Family Centred Care notes that, 'A patient is more than an aggregate of physical symptoms that need medicating or hospitalising but rather is someone who has strengths, expertise and resources. Acknowledging and tapping into these can empower both the patient and the health professional.'

This is true for all fields of medicine, including psychiatry and mental health. We need to move beyond the 'static model of doctor as giver, patient as receiver' and instead develop partnerships between patients, their families, carers and health professionals.

When someone is seriously mentally ill and unable to give a clear description of symptoms, family and carers are in the best position to provide health workers with information that is potentially lifesaving. I've spoken with many families and carers who are immensely frustrated that they are not heard or believed or taken seriously when they report that their loved one is becoming unwell and needs assessment and treatment. They know the patient best. They know what is usual and what is not and what is indicative of illness and relapse.

Patients also have skills and strengths. It hurts not to be respected or treated with dignity. Every human being has the same kind of heart. The same kinds of fears. The same need for connection.

28

Hot summer days. To improve general fitness I walk part of the way to and from work and ride my bike to the supermarket on weekends. The evenings are heavy with the day's heat and the nights hold the heat like they're breathing in but not out. I cold shower and reapply deodorant and still I sweat.

Climbing four flights of stairs to my office in the morning is grinding. My mind steps forward firmly but my body doesn't follow.

'I'm fucking wobbling instead of walking,' I say to Deborah. We laugh and then sigh. So I try harder – extend walking routes, ride faster, but the muscle fibres in my limbs have forgotten how to contract. Occasionally my legs jerk under the desk for no reason. Then I vomit twice on the way home from work, and when I stand up afterwards the world is spinning fast. It spins. Every time I re-open my eyes, it spins.

At home I ring a friend who lives just around the corner, Sharon, for help.

'Shaz, ish Kate. The leethum. Pees–'

'Kate, what the hell, I can't understand you.'

'If . . . to jive to the . . .'

'Hospital? Do you need the hospital?'

'Mmm.'

'Stay there. I'll be there.'

I slide to the floor, shuffle to the door; skitter down the stairs on all fours like a crab.

At the hospital the triage nurse and an orderly haul me somehow onto a bed and wheel me to a cubicle. Sharon goes outside for a smoke.

'What's been happening?' asks the registrar.

I hold out my hands, shaking, rattling hands. The registrar examines the muscle tone in my arms and legs, listens to my heartbeat, checks my eyes.

'How's your vision?'

I close my eyes and shake my head.

She takes a tendon hammer off a shelf and lightly taps both my patellar tendons (knee reflexes) and my legs shoot up like she's shot a current through them. She taps my left tendon and even my right leg reacts.

'Interesting,' she says. 'You've sure got some neurological thing going on here. Good that you came in.'

Someone else inserts an IV and takes blood. Before they return with the biochemistry and haematology results, the world recedes into a tunnel whose circumference narrows first to white and then to nothing.

When I wake up there's a brick on my chest. I try to move it away but it's attached via a number of wires to my skin. I lie in a stupor for several days. Sometimes I open my eyes to find friends and family sitting by the bed. I smile to them. Open my mouth, close it. Close my eyes. Open them again. They are gone.

'This is a portable ECG machine, linked up to a monitor in the clinical station,' says a nurse, checking the brick. 'Your lithium levels were way too high. Your kidneys aren't coping so well. You're in Cardiology because your heart is going too slowly.'

'Well. That sucks.' My glasses are on but everyone looks far away.

Voices leer in, drink the air and then sigh into the corners of the room. Four days after admission one of the nurses helps me sit up, slide to the edge of the bed and with a four-wheel walking frame I take a step. Another. A ten centimetre by ten centimetre long march to the toilet. Once there I need help to pull down my knickers and then I fall sideways off the seat. W.H Auden said, Art is born of humiliation. I would be happy, right now, to be forever and ever bereft of artistic inclination.

Litres of saline are pumped into my vascular system via the intravenous line and as a consequence the overload of lithium is excreted through my kidneys. The heart returns to a normal rhythm and the nervous system quietens.

'Don't forget to link up with a psychiatrist to re-start your lithium,' says the medical registrar as I'm discharged.

'Thanks,' I say to him. 'Fucking absurd drug,' I say to myself.

At home the books on the dark wood shelves seduce me – their secrets, the truths and lies. I love them for both the truths and the lies. I sit on the couch with a bottle of lithium tablets in my left hand and I sit for a long time and I don't know what to do.

The world is purer without the interference of such mind-altering substances. This particular mind-altering substance has made me very sick. On the other hand, without it there is the risk that I'll become very sick.

The next day I'm back at work, wobbling slightly and nauseated and I apologise to everyone and explain that I've been home with gastro. At lunchtime I go down to the medical library and pour over textbooks and journal articles on lithium – recommended doses, therapeutic concentrations, side effects, alternative treatments. A quarter of my previous daily dose is still within the recommended range. The lower the dose, the fewer adverse effects. This is worthy of a personal experiment.

Hypothesis: on the new dose of lithium I'll remain well, think and concentrate better and reduce the risk of toxicity. Perfect.

Weeks pass and I note only subtle tremor in my arms and legs, less extreme thirst, less nausea and no diarrhoea. I feel stronger, I have more energy and I'm more alive to the world.

Mog, the new foster kitten, is phytophilous. Succulents and cacti, previously in pots on the living room window-ledge, are this morning dug up, dismembered and scattered over the floorboards. Her cat toys – balls and furry mice – are untouched. From the courtyard she brings in leaves and twigs and purple ivy flowers and deposits them on my bed. Every day more foliage: bits of bark, grass, new shoots, tiny white flowers, long lines of creeper, green leaves, brown leaves, seedpods. When I open the front door, home from work, she trills like a bird. She is afraid of birds. There are no circumstances under which I can relinquish such an amazingly gorgeous and original feline, so I ring the animal shelter to arrange adoption.

The big fat cat (Her Royal Greyness) is not impressed with the new addition to our family. She glares at Mog every morning, grey tail fluffed, heavy-breathing. Then she growls, a low rumble that builds in volume and pitch as it moves through her body. She chew-growls, purr-growls, even snore-growls. Oh she glares.

At the next session with Winsome I sit on the couch next to a bright pink elephant called 'No Longer Taking The Prescribed Dose Of Lithium'. The elephant is quiet and still throughout, his leathery pink skin just touching my thigh. The softest, finest touch. About which I say nothing.

Afterwards, back in the car, I lean on the steering wheel and turn the music up and write the justification out like a testament—

This is a private experiment.

It's my brain. It's my research into the neurochemistry of my brain.

I do not need permission – I'm not five years old.

No-one has the right to dictate what I put in my body or when or how much. Enough damage done.

There is potential for discovery. A leap. A passage through.

There's something about the evening sky tonight. It is speaking . . . no, it is singing. Each second the light changes, bleeding out colour. A painter would need to work fast, melding rose and orange with dream and perfume and infinitesimal shifts in hue. How is it that this transition from bright to dark retains its beauty with every tick and blink?

I inhale it and it fills me and I weep.

Oh god, am I effectively cured?

At night I walk. At night I read about Ötzi the Iceman, who lived in the Austrian Alps 5000 years ago. At night Ötzi enters my room, my bed, my head.

He is great – this Shaman, masked with the head of a bison. He is strung with copper amulets, stone and marble, and chants his prayers before an altar with the residue of gold on his brow. While the rest harvest the dance – though they move in a trance the sacrifice is real – women sit and sway with the chanting, their breaths are hums engraved with teeth.

Four chiefs in an arc frame the fires, and on the altar table carved grooves gather the edges like garlands around a feast of horned beasts—those that drew granite and onyx, those that drew breath white in the night, whose eyes held quicksilver when the fires burned orange and bloody in the black sky.

And a river of ice: gray, surreal, crawls from behind the alpine arc, gnaws at the feet of the Ötztal Alps, and carves anew the valley floor. Mountain bogs strung with ice-pollen enclose a death in this pale space. Men with dagger and plaited scabbard wait, as the Shaman chants his prayers; whorls of stone blur in their heads.

Where the sun-symbols, radiant even in stone, meet and meld, there the crucible is set down on the altar. Boar husks, the severed antlers of a stag covered with birch fungus and blue-bloomed berries, are given over to a Neolithic death. All is covered with fire and prayer, till the echoes sing of fire and prayer, and the residue of seven thousand human skulls rattle their jaws over the walls of Val Venosta.

This is the time for studying music theory and astronomy. I love the words of music: portamento, glissando, richochet, spiccato – a kind of onomatopeic poem. I buy textbooks and notebooks and workbooks and star charts. My parents buy me a Schmidt-Cassegrain telescope for Christmas. It has eight inches of light-gathering aperture for viewing the carnival of deep space and the surface of Jupiter and Saturn's rings.

We take it outside, polar-align and set it to the celestial co-ordinates of the moon. The moon has a long association with insanity. The words lunacy and lunatic and loony are derived from the Roman goddess of the moon, Luna. There is no scientific evidence to support the belief that admissions to psychiatric hospitals, crimes or suicides increase during a full moon. Still, observing the moon through the telescope in its first quarter, with the low sun casting shadows that define lava plains and craters and white mountain ranges, I'm expanded and gripped and flung apart and I feel infinitely small and finite.

Oh god, I am effectively cured.

On my bedroom wall I pin a poster of the Hebrew aleph-bet. It's a colourful list of the Hebrew letters (. . . ג, ב, א) and their Latin transliteration (aleph, bet, gimel . . .). Here in my room is the sacred language of The Torah, The Holy Bible, of Jerusalem. Like all Semitic languages, Hebrew is written from right to left, without vowels. My brain takes a few days to adjust, a few weeks to recognise the letters automatically and begin to interpret words. It's glorious.

At work, right earphone plugged into Schubert's String Quintet in C major opus 163, I read from Hebrew language textbooks piled on my lap under the desk.

'Ani rotsah levaker beYerushalayim (בירושלים) bevakasha,' I whisper to myself. 'Ani rotsah lalekhet la'ir haatika.'

I book a flight to Tel Aviv via Paris, departure date in three months. To prepare for travelling in Israel, I answer my work colleagues' questions in half-Hebrew, half-English, which they seem to find irritating, and oddly, none of them is interested in either my translations or explanations of pronunciation and nuance.

Showering two or three times a day is for the sound of water on my skin and the gossamer feel of a layer of cleanser between my hands and breasts. The scents of orange oil and frankincense baptise the steam and rise. It occurs to me that the connection between Scent and Essence is consummated in Essential, expanding into Elixir and Substance, contracting into Core and Heart.

So I trawl through pharmacies and skin care shops, studying ingredient lists and lingering over advertised efficacies: cleansing and peeling and refining and soothing and smoothing and hydrating and moisturising. I buy six kinds of facial scrub, which I mix together into a strange green-brown paste. I buy enzyme peels, tonics and toners and serums, mineral masques, night gels with moonflower and grapefruit extract. Some particularly exotic products are, via the internet, sent direct from Paris and the Dead Sea. I line tubes and bottles in rows on the bathroom floor and apply them to my face in a riot of layers. Over time my skin reddens and flakes, and then weeps.

At work I divide the day into ten minute segments: ten minutes of work, ten minutes of Hebrew, ten minutes grappling with the physics of neutron stars, ten minutes listening to a recording of *Under Milk-wood* through one ear bud so I can still hear the phone. Given that my nutritional status is poor, I buy a bottle of multivitamins and take thirty tablets one day, thirty the next. Done. Oranges, derivates of the sun, provide sustenance while I crystallise a new theory of evolution.

At the Esplanade Hotel in St Kilda, it's live percussion and rap. Five young men on a variety of drums and one young woman rapping about hell and the devil and Jesus and shit. The music gets right into my heart and veins and runs like blood all through me. I have to dance so I dance with the beat of the surdo and the sunset, with the sun – which is flirting with the clouds and sea, teasing and then leaving.

Once home I jog down to the local park and throw my shoes into a maple tree and dance in the dark. The grass is breathing, breathing under my bare feet.

'Kate, what the hell are you doing out here?' Naava is standing in the middle of the park, hands on hips, the top of her head halo-like where it's caught by the moon.

'Patterns in the stars!' I shout.

'Shhh . . . you've left all your doors and windows open.'

'What?'

'Come on. Come on, please.'

'No.'

'Where are your shoes?'

'No idea. Sorry, oh my god, that's so funny!'

'It's not bloody funny.'

'Did you see the coronal loops of the sun?'

'No.'

'Millions of brilliance, rays from Ra—'

'You can't stay out here. Come home. Please.'

'Piss off, honey, I'm communing with a woman and a man and the sun before it bursts.'

'Come and have a drink with me.'

'Yippee, right-oh.'

We walk up the drive. Lights are on, doors and windows open, Jane's Addiction blaring.

'We're going to see Jenny in the morning,' says Naava.

'Groovy.'

Naava sleeps on the couch downstairs. I sit up all night reading Gerard Manley Hopkins out loud to the cats.

'It just came to me like magic – an epiphany!' I explain to Jenny in the morning. 'This could be a world first, another step forward for Homo sapiens, think of all the money I'm going to save and no more time wasted shopping for food.'

'What are you talking about?' asks Jenny.

Naava opens out her hands, palms up.

'I'm a heliotrope! I've got sunshine in my veins!' I say.

'Can you tell me what's been happening Naava?' asks Jenny.

Naava talks quietly. I can't hear her properly because of the buzzing in the room. As she talks, Jenny opens a drawer in her desk and pulls out a sheet of tablets.

I roll my eyes. 'Here we go.'

'Risperidone,' says Jenny. 'Soluble.' Meaning the tablets will dissolve in my mouth without water.

I like Jenny and I respect her, so I take the tablet. It tastes like peppermint. Jenny gives Naava the packet of risperidone. 'I'd like you to have another one tonight,' she says to me. 'Okay?' Then she looks at Naava. 'And I'll notify the Crisis Assessment Team.'

'Cats, cats, cats,' I say.

In the evening, Zoë comes over after work. There is a tiny segment of my mind that recognises that Zoë and Naava are worried, and it appreciates that they are here. The rest of my mind is intent, fluid, pure. The Crisis Assessment Team arrives at 9 p.m. in their generic white car. I sit up straight on the floor of the living room and expound the chaos theory of evolution, 'Change can happen in bursts, it's not always sequential, if DNA mutates in positive ways, then as trees grow new branches, there are infinite possibilities. Right?'

Silence.

'Okay,' I whisper to my feet, rocking back and forward, 'Fractals are unanswerable questions. Fractals are unanswerable questions.'

One of the team goes outside to make a phone call, the other says, 'We're going to take you into hospital, Kate, your mood is elevated and you're pretty pre-occupied and Jenny tells us that you haven't been eating properly, is that right?'

'I've got sunshine in my veins.'

Zoë packs a bag of clothes. I add notebooks and coloured pencils, the *Norton Anthology of Poetry* in two volumes, a Hebrew-English dictionary and a bottle of gin. Zoë takes out the bottle of gin.

On the way to the hospital the streetlights penetrate my irises and fingerprint my retinae.

'Why aren't you eating?' asks Graham, one of the consultant psychiatrists on the inpatient unit, in the morning.

'I'm generating energy from the sun. You remember the equation for photosynthesis: carbon dioxide plus water mixed with chlorophyll and sunlight equals glucose and oxygen.'

'You are not a plant, Kate.'

'I know, I KNOW, that's precisely why this could be an evolutionary event. Breathe with me. I'll breathe your carbon dioxide. You breathe my oxygen. A cosmic force is slouching towards Bethlehem, just like Yeats said.'

'Are you hungry?'

'Hungry is for ephemerals.'

Graham turns to Brenda, the registrar. 'What dose have we got her on?'

'Olanzapine 20 mg and lithium 1000.'

'Right.' He stands up. 'See you tomorrow.'

I go back out into the courtyard with my notebooks, rolling my jeans up, taking off my jumper and shirt and stretching out on one of the wooden benches next to Claude in the sun. Claude is in his early thirties, tall, very pale. Thin. He's wearing tight black jeans and a black shirt with long sleeves and a collar. His black fringe covers his eyes.

'The government says it will halve the rate of homelessness in ten years, and they will too, because half of the homeless will be dead in ten years,' he says, sitting with his hands clasped over his head, blue veins communicating that universal thing – despair.

'Drum sticks aren't ecological. They're an extenuating circumstance. Hands are all you need. Though it is up to interpretation – no-one has exclusive rights,' I reply.

'What?' he says, looking up.

'Extenuating circumstances. Are you being circological?'

'You said ecological.'

'No, I meant the complete opposite.'

'Huh?'

'Extension of the hand, that's it. Here's a message from Jesus, can you divine me? Put your hands in mine, I'll divine you; I'll divine your thoughts.'

Claude shakes his head.

'Are you speaking figuratively?' he asks after a while.

'Regardless, we are in fact, seven-point-stars, all of us in here. Did you know, technically, the piano is a percussion instrument because it has hammers? Then again, it has strings. It has keys! Is that it?'

'You're such a bullshitter,' says Claude. He stands up and walks away and sits down over the other side of the courtyard.

'You know what?' I shout. 'My mouth has its own little brain – it's a very small brain, not much more than a brainstem really, and it doesn't have an off-switch.'

And then I start to cry though I'm not at all sad. Even my eyelids are sunburnt.

Tadiwa is Zimbabwean. She's my regular contact nurse.

'Are most of your family back home, Tadiwa?' I ask.

'Yes,' she says. Even her yes is lilting. 'In Harare.'

'Is it hard?'

'Yes.'

'Are they safe?'

'Well . . . it is in God's hands.'

'Something has happened to time,' I say to Zoë and Deborah. 'It's stopped following the rules of second, minute, hour. It runs backwards, then races forwards, swallowing the ticks in between before we have a chance to live in them. Have you noticed?'

'No, not really, Kate.'

'Never mind, I'm writing it all down, keeping tabs. Later my notes will be given in evidence.' I pull out my notebooks and flick through the tatty pages. 'See?'

Zoë and Deborah smile and nod.

'When did you last eat?' asks Brenda one morning.

'No idea oh my god energy I reckon I'm conductive connect me up to some copper wire and I'll generate electricity alchemy was all about transforming lesser metals into gold Isaac Newton was an alchemist this is the elixir of life round round rock clock dans les veines de Pan mettaient un universe that's Rimbaud for you he totally got it unlike you lot Christ have you no souls there's a fire angel out in the courtyard maybe you need to burn up a bit to discover something that actually matters my jumper in tatters elastic will stretch so far then it shatters my cat's tail has rhythm like Emily Dickinson—'

'Shut up for a second, please,' says Graham.

I glare at him and get out my notebooks and some coloured pencils. I can't find my fountain pen or my stash of coffee nor my bottle of gin but I have my notebooks.

'It's been two weeks. You need to start eating,' says Graham.

'When you grasp the complexity of the situation you won't make suggestions,' I reply.

'You have twenty-four hours in which to change to your mind,' says Graham calmly. 'If not, we're transferring you to HDU and we'll insert a nasogastric tube.'

I walk out of the room, back to the courtyard and lie down on the concrete. Sunshine and carbon dioxide.

'I've got Vanilla Ensure or Resource Fruit,' says Tadiwa, coming into my room the following morning, holding a can in one hand and a tetra-pak in the other.

'Will it save your family?'

'Pardon?'

'If I drink this.'

'I'm not sure about that. But you're going to end up with a tube down your throat if you don't drink it.'

'Will it save your family?'

'No, Kate.'

I shake my head.

'Vanilla Ensure or Resource Fruit?' asks Tadiwa, the morning after.

'Will it save your family?'

'Well it will help me, and I'm part of my family.'

'Yeah?'

'Yeah. I don't want you to have a tube.' She smiles then, full of light, and she pulls the lid off the can of Ensure and holds it out and I take it and drink some and it's like condensed milk.

'Finish it?' says Tadiwa.

'Enough.'

'For me?'

I drink it slowly. It's so glutinous and sweet I want to vomit but I drink it.

'Good on you, I'll be back at lunchtime,' says Tadiwa.

'Now Kate, you're at risk of re-feeding syndrome,' says Brenda in the afternoon.

'Re-what syndrome?'

'Re-feeding syndrome. Your electrolyte and glucose levels in the blood could change very rapidly once you're eating again. Your heart can go into a dangerous kind of arrhythmia.'

'Yep,' I say. I'm fascinated by Tadiwa's necklace, its Byzantine rose-gold is whispering stories.

'So, we're going to do a blood test twice a day for a few days.'

'Yep.'

'Are you hearing me?'

'For they will inherit the earth,' I whisper.

'Good,' Brenda says.

In the evening I sit next to Claude in the common room. The people on television are high-pitched and the women are dressed like lorikeets.

'The Disability Support Pension keeps us below the poverty line but there's always millions of tax payers' dollars to promote sport,' says Claude.

I get up and shake his hands – first right, then left. 'Gentleman,' I say, 'You speak the truth. I have to go and write that down verbatim.'

'Claude, here are your meds for tonight,' says Maree, one of the nursing staff.

'I'm just trying to outrun the devil and the churches are all locked,' says Claude.

Maree waits.

'No such thing as sanctuary. No such thing as refuge,' he says to his feet.

'Okay, well take these, please.' Maree has a tiny plastic cup with several tablets in it, and some water.

'How do you expect to unlock a unique mind with the same damn key?' I ask Maree. 'Why would the same key fit into every brain, when each houses the central nervous system, the mind with all its idiosyncrasies and even the soul?' I rock back on my heels. 'No wonder this medication is crap. No wonder there are so many side effects. Medication should be tailored to individuality. House keys and car keys are – why do you keep shoving stuff that is blunt as hammers down our throats?'

'There's always ECT,' says Maree dryly.

'ECT is worse. It's a fucking jackhammer. No, that's not right – it's a sanctioned version of the electric chair.'

'Have youz got any perfume?' asks another patient. 'Do I stink or what? Oh I feel sick, all I can smell is smoke. Where's Shane? See how red my shoes are? Hey! Have youz got any perfume or not?'

'Yeah,' I say. 'In my room.'

'Can I have this?' she asks.

'Yeah.'

I sit on the bed. How have I come to be here, useless as a baby, equally reliant, equally incompetent. Equally? Less even?

Mania is initially as seductive as a snort of coke, a first orgasm, a religious epiphany. The world fizzes. And the illness progresses.

One is gripped, vice-like, by irritability and wild risk-taking with money or sex or drugs or alcohol or all four together. One is swallowed up into the guts of a chimera, wherein lie delusions and hallucinations and chaos.

The day before I'm discharged, Deborah picks me up and we drive to a small bluestone church in Fitzroy. The Anglo-Catholic incense – is it frankincense? Myrrh? It smells like cloves and cardamom. The choir starts to sing 'Spem in alium'. . . I have never put my hope in any other but in you. 'Spem in alium' is a motet written for forty individual parts by Thomas Tallis. The choir sings in the round – spaced out along the walls and the front and back of the church so the music passes from north to south and east to west or sometimes south to east to north and then west. Voices like syrup, like black ice reflecting, like autumn and clouds and the dusky sky – love and sorrow and grace and love. The polyphonic sound touches and lips and falls and runs and rises and my body dissolves; I disappear altogether, all there is and all there will ever be is this – this music. Spem in alium nunquam habui præter in te, Deus Israel.

'Love this music,' Deborah says when the choir finishes. 'Love you.'

'Love this music,' I say. 'Love you.'

The poetry anthology, the Hebrew dictionary and notebooks and now-too-big clothes are packed to come home with Zoë and Naava and I, along with a bottle of lithium tablets and some olanzapine.

We debrief on the couch.

'How long was I in hospital?'

'Three weeks,' says Zoë.

'The front fender has almost fallen off my car. And the driver-side door panel's all warped. Jesus. What did I do?'

'We don't know.'

I begin to weep. The weeping regresses into guttural sobs. Then I breathe, suck it all up inside and am still. Parsha (The Pygmy Tiger) curls onto my chest. I put my hands around her abdomen – lightly, and watch my fingers spread a little apart with her breath and I can feel the beat of her heart. Ah, this thing called life.

'So my carefully constructed hypothesis, that I'd remain well on the lowest possible dose of lithium, has been disproved,' I say to Winsome a week later. 'Fuck it.'

'Kate,' she says, 'Surely it is clear now that you can't make these kinds of decisions about medication on your own. You must do so in partnership with a clinician.'

I sigh.

'It's essential.'

'How the hell do I find a psychiatrist who understands *primum non nocere*? The *Yellow Pages*?'

'What about asking Jenny for a recommendation?'

I consider. 'Okay. I can do that.'

Then I catch the train into work for a meeting with my manager. Though I've already arranged the next four weeks as annual leave, they'll add to the previous four weeks of leave without pay. Two months in total during which my colleagues are left to manage my workload as well as their own.

I can't face them. I'm gut-sick about it. I'm not well enough. Guilt. I'll never work again. I have to work again. Shame. It is impossible to be more unreliable. I love my work friends. I've let them down. It's an illness. Jesus.

Shame.

Diana, my manager, is calm and realistic, and (oh-thank-you-universe) she doesn't sack me or suggest I resign. I tell her I'm struggling with a 'mental health problem'. She ingests this quietly and doesn't pry. We develop a return to work plan. I apologise to my colleagues a thousand times and assist with the problems they've had while I've been away as best I can.

'There is a difference between intellectually knowing something – and integrating, absorbing and owning it,' says Winsome the following week. 'Does that make some sense?'

'Yeah, it does.'

'We both know you've had the intellectual knowledge about your illness for some time.'

I nod.

'But you haven't owned it.'

I frown, wriggle my feet, look at the floor, out the window, back at the floor. Then I look at Winsome.

'True,' I say.

'And now?'

'I think . . . I mean I know . . . I have a mental illness. And that my old, carefully constructed reality was, in fact, false – I mean, to the point of delusional.'

'Yes.'

Suddenly here we are, me and it – the illness – face to face in Winsome's office. It's ugly, an unhealing wound. Blind and violent. I stare it down.

'I accept that I'll have to take medication for the rest of my life.'

'Because?'

'If I stop taking it, I lose touch with reality. My thinking goes off, and then my behaviour goes off.'

'What's the worst thing that could happen?'

'Suicide obviously . . . and that I might hurt someone – hurt someone I love.'

'And apart from medication?'

'Taking responsibility. For all the bits of my life.' I pause and then smile. 'Especially the dysfunctional bits, right?'

'Yes,' Winsome smiles back.

Together we draw up a list of early warning signs, subtle changes in affect (mood), thinking, perception and behaviour.

'What's the very first thing you notice?' Winsome asks.

'Heightened sensitivity,' I say. 'To sound – the loudness of someone's voice or the pitch of a musical note or a particular kind of sound; sometimes I can listen to an oboe but not a clarinet. And to light, especially dusk, and to temperature – hot water or cold wind. Later on any extremes of sound or sudden bright light are physically painful – like being hit with a taser.'

The medical journals and practice guidelines report that up to 70 per cent of people experience early warning signs over a period of one to four weeks prior to relapse into an acute illness like mania or severe depression or psychosis.

'After that?' Winsome asks.

'Sensitivity becomes intensity becomes . . . menacing. This inexplicable and pervasive dread.'

'And then?'

'The nightmares start and my sleep pattern changes and my mood changes – either melancholic or kind of elevated and buzzing. To combat all this, in the past, I'd start drinking a lot of whisky to anaesthetise myself.'

Some early warning signs are common among people with a particular illness but many are unique. A relapse signature is a list, usually time-dependent, of an individual's early warning signs.

'Season change is risky for mood change,' I say. 'Especially from summer to autumn – those cooler, shorter evenings, and from winter to spring – the warmer, longer evenings.'

'Why?'

'I don't know . . . maybe it's about light and melatonin. Maybe it's the idea of transition. Whatever the reason, it's a trigger.'

My relapse signature continues with irritability and restlessness or a weird heaviness in the chest. Sometimes concentration deteriorates.

'Other times,' I say to Winsome, 'it's like I've got two brains.'

'This is when you must ask for help,' she says.

I nod. 'Because obsessive thinking follows, and then strange preoccupations and chain smoking and suspiciousness. And I'm starting to lose insight – around the edges.'

Winsome writes everything down in red on her whiteboard so I can't hide from it.

'What happens next?'

'This is hard, to you know, to say out loud.'

We pause for a while.

'Shit,' I say. 'Okay . . . flight of ideas, visions, serious insomnia and neglect – neglect of the things that matter like family and my wonderful friends and work responsibilities and home and well, me.'

'You know, Kate, the earlier we intervene the better, for reducing severity and shortening the duration of relapse. Yes?'

'Yes.'

'Okay. What next?'

'The ends of the earth. Usually I'll stop eating but I'll be drinking a lot of scotch or vodka. All I can hear are command hallucinations, *do this . . .*'

Based on my relapse signature, we draw up an action plan in exactly the same way asthmatics and diabetics have an action plan. We talk about the importance of seeking help before I begin to lose insight and about reality testing. That is, checking in with someone I trust about obsessive thoughts. Or sudden new ideas. Or changes in mood that are unrelated to external events.

'And medication?'

'Hah! No self-medication. I'll make an appointment with Jenny.'

'Do you trust Jenny?'

'Yes.'

'That's the most important thing,' Winsome says. Then she says, 'You have ownership of this illness. You have ownership and control.'

I roll my eyes. 'It's only taken me ten years of trying every kind of medication . . . and therapy.'

'Now travel safely and keep well and we'll continue the discussion when you're back home.'

'Be'seder. Merci, Madame.'

29

At 2 a.m. I take a taxi to the airport and board a flight to Paris. Thanks to the sedating effect of olanzapine, I sleep for the first half of the flight and then read till we land at Charles de Gaulle.

Rising up from the Metro. Heartbeat. Flush. Breath.

Here is the Jardin du Luxembourg on one side and on the other, ah – the beautiful buildings of the Sorbonne. Here perhaps, walked Sartre and de Beauvoir. I slide my backpack to the ground and sit on it. This is about experiencing the world as a newborn – free of the people in my head and the associated paranoia and magical thinking. Free to absorb the world exactly as it is.

My little hotel is in the Quartier Latin. I find a cafe near the Panthéon and drink coffee in the sunshine and people walking by half-smile at me or half-frown and I realise I'm grinning.

On Île de la Cité, amongst the buildings of the Palais de Justice is La Sainte Chapelle. The gothic ceiling of the lower chapel, a blue-heaven canopy, reaches down with generous gilt arms to support the floor. The upper third of the walls are stained glass and are beautiful – and whet the appetite. I climb the single flight of stairs.

Heartbeat. Flush. Breath.

There are no structural supports inside the chapel; nothing impedes my gaze no matter where I cast my eyes.

And nothing is in shadow.

The room is aflame. The current of light. The veins of colour. The enormous flowering. Here is a thing envisioned and created by a group of people 750 years ago that, I think, rivals the beauty of nature. It's a breath from alive. The stone floor is undulating, dimpled around the perimeter, so many feet.

I walk over to Île St Louis past the formidable walls of Notre-Dame, onto the right bank of the Seine and then into the Marais for an early bistro dinner.

'Vous désirez?' asks the waiter.

'Est-ce que vous avez une carte en Anglais?'

'Non.'

'Oh. Okay. Um . . .' The menu is hand-written. Finally I find a word I understand. 'Steak tartare, s'il vous plaît.'

The waiter nods and smiles and ten minutes later I'm presented with a plate of chilled, finely chopped and seasoned raw steak, garnished with raw onion and a raw egg yolk. The waiter smiles again, and yes, I know exactly what he is thinking.

In the Musée D'Orsay are paintings by Klimt and Gauguin and Pissarro. This is pretty close to heaven. The queue out the front is long. I stand on one leg, swap to the other, look at the trees. People are chatting and laughing as they wait and suddenly I'm terribly alone. But once inside, the art up close is more astonishing than I'd imagined. In one room are thirteen paintings by Vincent Van Gogh, including a *Portrait de l'artiste* and *La nuit étoilée*. Oh, those very brush strokes!

With my last two days I visit the Musée Rodin for his bronze sculpture, *The Thinker* and Montmartre for the Espace Dali, whose work is, in his own words, an expression of 'the associations and interpretations of delirious phenomena.' Mostly I'm reminded of psychosis, in the sense that I wonder if his interpretation of the world is bizarre enough to be impenetrable and unreachable by a majority of sane folk.

In the Marais district along rue de Thorigny is the elegant, aristocratic mansion, l'hôtel Salé, now home to the Musée Picasso. This artist catapults me out of myself, swings me around near the ceiling, flings me to the stars, steps on me hard, drags me through the blackness of hell and sets me weeping before the simplest line drawing.

The next morning I lug my backpack onto the train from Paris central to Charles de Gaulle airport. On the flight to Israel is a group of American evangelicals, all with bibles and nametags and hats. They're touring the Christian Holy Land in ten days – Sea of Galilee, Bethlehem, the Via Dolorosa, Church of the Holy Sepulchre and Gethsemane. The plane lands in Tel Aviv in the late afternoon and Naava is meeting me in the arrivals hall. The hall is huge, packed with family groups, kids with flowers and Israeli flags and black-suited, black-hatted Charedi men and I can't see her anywhere. The awareness that I miss her and I miss Zoë and my family hits suddenly in the guts. Eventually we find each other after an hour of wandering in circles and wrap each other up like we've been apart for years.

We take a highway bus through the steep, winding, bone-coloured Judean hills. It is warm; the sky blazes blue. No clouds. We pass several flat-topped towns and the occasional date palm. Through a ravine and over a hill and here before us—

Yerushalayim. al-Quds. City of Gold. Jerusalem.

Naava is staying with relatives and I'm booked into a convent in the Muslim Quarter of the Old City. Jerusalem is divided in many ways and on many levels. One – denoting history – is the demarcation between modern East and West Jerusalem, and the Old City, which itself is divided into the same four quarters laid out by the Romans in 135 CE.

Along the stone paths of the Old City I walk with Chassidic men, IDF soldiers carrying Tavor assault rifles, Russian tourists, secular Israelis, men shrouded in white keffiyeh and women in hijab and long dresses. Here is a donkey and some boys on bicycles, here are women sitting cross-legged on the side of the road selling mint and parsley. Now the smell of Arabic coffee and cardamom and sweet nargilah tobacco.

I turn into the Via Dolorosa (Way of Sorrow) – the path Jesus took from Gethsemane to Golgotha. The front door of the convent is the tallest, broadest, strongest-looking dark wooden door I've ever seen, with a thick metal knocker. I knock.

Like many buildings in Israel, the flat convent roof is a place to gather for tea and conversation or for silent contemplation. I bring with me a copy of the Bible I found in my room. The roof overlooks the Temple Mount to the south, the Christian Quarter of the Old City to the west and rising up to the southeast is the Mount of Olives. Everywhere domes and minarets and church spires and stone crosses and aerials and antennae and electrical wires.

I read from the Psalms and watch the light fade. There's a slight breeze and the air smells of dust and cedar. A flock of grey and white doves weaves and rises and falls and rises above the roofs towards the sun and just as they reach its lower pole, they turn as if faced with God and burned, and dive as one back to earth.

'How beautiful you are my darling! Oh, how beautiful! Your eyes are doves.' Song of Songs.

This city is more than history and architecture and culture and religion. It is intensity of feeling – it's on people's faces, it has moulded into their bodies and permeated the stone streets. It's everywhere, this thing I'm searching and searching for – meaning.

Dawn.

'Allahu Akbar, Allahu Akbar,

Ash-had an la ilaha illa llah . . .'

A local Muezzin calls the Islamic faithful to prayer; his melismatic voice stretches out over the Old City. I get up from the narrow bed overhung with a crucifix and re-align the scratchy blankets and take the medication with water and walk down El Wad Road to the Jewish Quarter for an Israeli breakfast and sweet mint tea.

In the Christian Quarter further west is the Church of the Holy Sepulchre, visited by 16 centuries of Christian pilgrims. Inside, it's more a collection of chapels, dark and cool. Electric lanterns and candles provide light. The floor is mostly marble and the walls and stairs are limestone. The voices and feet of tourist groups echo up into the vaulted roof and fall down again like rain.

People are kneeling in prayer before the Twelfth Station of the Cross – the site of the crucifixion. Over the bare rock is a marble altar, and above that, a life-size statue of Jesus. Surrounding him are oil lamps and candles and a reflecting relief in silver and gold that makes my eyes water.

The peripheral chapels are still and sombre and grey-brown dark. I run my palms over lines of crosses etched into the walls – some date back to the time of the crusades. I close my eyes and breathe and my heart runs, blood runs and fills and deepens.

Later Naava and I explore Ir David – the archaeological site outside the walls of the Old City that is, says Yael our guide, the location of Biblical King David's Palace. Suddenly I'm standing on land that has had significance for people for over 3000 years, and whose ownership remains fraught. The continuing excavations are encroaching on the Palestinian town of Silwan.

We have dinner in the Muslim Quarter. Naava and I are the only women sitting on tiny chairs on the side of the street, drinking coffee, black and strong and flavoured with cardamom. We order a nargilah. The coals have been burning for hours so the smoke is at once thick and sweet and . . . the world is spinning.

We stretch out our legs under the table. The men stare for a while and then resume their conversations.

'This is amazing,' I say.

'It is,' says Naava. She looks like she's going to melt into the chair.

'I mean this part of Jerusalem . . . being here . . . right at this spot right at this moment. Here with you. Amazing.'

The next day is Holocaust Remembrance Day. I walk up the narrow, winding road to the Mount of Olives. Its slopes have been used as a place of burial for millennia. It is here that the Messiah will first appear before passing through the Golden Gate to the Temple Mount. It is from here that Jesus ascended to Heaven. And here is the sunrise over the Old City, flushing the pale limestone tombs, blushing the city walls and polishing the Dome of The Rock from burnished to bright gold. Oh Yerushalayim, the light, the light.

The sirens start at 10 a.m. A steady wail, a cry of pain, higher in pitch than a lament. The cars and buses and trucks on Jaffa Road stop. People turn off their engines and get out and stand still and silent in the middle of the road and bow their heads. I stand and bow my head. The sirens keen for two minutes, after which, people continue quietly on their way.

This land is sacred to all three monotheistic religions and to Sufis, Druze, Baha'i and Bedouins. The land has been fought over by Egyptians, Greeks, Romans, Ottomans, Crusaders, Turks, Napoleon and the British. There are communities here from Ethiopia, North

ירושלים.
אמן.
(Amen).
My heart.
לב.

Where Jerusalem ends,
the desert begins.

Just the muddy-red + mustard
sides of the ravine and the sandy
ground under my feet.
No wind. No voices between
Bethlehem and Hebron + Bi'er Sheva.
Think/Feel → we all have
different sacred stuff, it both
nourishes and feeds.

(not mine)
אֵלֶּך, אַרְצָה...

heart, head, land. The balance
of light. Lucency. It must have
been a vision under all skies.

the treasures
here in the desert.
The sand so soft. The light.

Africa, the Mediterranean, East and West Europe, Yemen, Iraq, North and South America. There are endless questions. There is absolute certainty and absolute unease. I'm expanded and gripped and flung apart and I feel again as I do observing the stars: infinitely small and finite.

'Pray for the peace of Jerusalem: may those who love you be secure. May there be peace within your walls.' Psalm 122.

Where Jerusalem ends, the desert begins – the Judean desert to the east, the Negev to the south. I'll travel on my own for a week and then meet Naava in Eilat by the Red Sea.

Everyone drives fast in Israel. This is my first time driving on the right side of the road in a left-hand-drive car. It's crazy. Somehow I memorise enough of the map to allow me to concentrate on avoiding hitting anything till I reach the wide, straight Number 6 Highway.

There are Bedouin tents hunched into the hills, rusting cars and sheet metal, rubbish piles, donkeys and goats. Large towns become smaller towns, then a Kibbutz with date palm plantations and occasional bursts of wildflowers. Then desert – dusky rock dotted with army-green shrubs. The 'lone and level sands' stretching far away.

Amid the occasional bank of army tanks and the desert and the deepening light, I find Mitzpeh Ramon: a town perched on the rim of the largest naturally formed crater in the world, and one of the best locations for desert hiking.

At sunrise I pack a good topographic map, compass, plenty of water, fruit and a hat. I'm wearing long loose pants and a long-sleeved shirt.

Walking along the wadi – the dry riverbed. No trees. No plant-life. No animals, no insects. Just the mustard and muddy-red sides of the ravine and the sandy ground under my feet.

No wind.

If I stop walking, absolute silence.

Then four jet fighter aircraft in formation. The lower thud of Apache helicopters.

Absolute silence.

30

Zoë and Naava and I talk when I get home about the business of a psychiatrist. It can't hurt, they say. Oh yes it can, I think, but it's also possible that Zoë and Naava and Winsome are right– psychiatrists have the specialised knowledge and experience to best manage long term illnesses like mine. So I visit Jenny and get a referral to Martin, who works in the private sector, at one of those bright, shiny private clinics.

Martin is very contained, very measured, like he has packed his real self up and left it outside the door of his consulting room. The bit that's left is probably unshockable, and as such he is safe from the vicissitudes of his patients – our pain and our neediness. We stride or slink through his door, our eyes and our faces shouting, 'Just fix it, please, just make it go away, just explain what the hell we're doing here – on this earth, PLEASE.' And he does none of these things of course, he sits and waits and lets us pour ourselves out like vomit on the floor and we sit in it, mired in our own filth, and then we have only half an hour to swallow it all up inside our- selves and somehow get to our feet and walk like normal people back out into the world.

Winsome and I continue the discussion about illness and wellness, and reflect on the tension between reality, rationality and the world of madness.

'For so long death has been the only salvation. That's hard to reconcile,' I say. 'I'm really . . . just plain sad that I've been unwell for . . . how long? Fifteen years. There have been times of reprieve but the longest they've ever lasted until now is eighteen months.'

'Psychology is a forensic process in a way,' Winsome says. 'Requiring the development of several hypotheses that can be tested over time.'

'Yeah, I see how that works.'

'It took a long time for me to understand, at least in part, what was going on inside your head.'

'I'm sorry.'

'Not at all. In the beginning our work was about me containing you in a non-judgmental space for day-to-day problem solving and crisis management.'

'Yes.'

'Because it is impossible to engage in the deep and complex process of any other kind of therapy when you are acutely unwell.' She pauses. 'Now you know that the mental illness is only one part of you; it is not the whole of you.'

'You think?'

'I'll say it again. The mental illness is only one part of you; it is not the whole of you. And mental illness can be managed.'

I look at her.

'When you were sixteen the crazy stuff started and all your energy went into managing that and there was nothing left to establish a normal and integrated sense of self. It was fifteen years of total chaos really, wasn't it?'

'Yes,' I put my head in my hands.

'Fifteen years of dysfunctional thinking . . .'

'Yes.' Muffled.

'Dread and terror and blackness . . .'

'Yes.'

'Avowed self-loathing . . .'

'Yes.'

'None of which was logical in any way.'

I look up. Winsome looks at me.

'None of which was logical in any way.'

She pauses.

'What is going to keep you well, Kate?'

'Balance,' I say.

Martin and I meet monthly. He doesn't say much. We both maintain a kind of professional reserve. I'm afraid of Martin. He has the power to lock me up, to deprive me of liberty and independence. He has the power to say, 'Kate is mad.' And if he does so, people will believe him. Certifying someone under the Mental Health Act is a last resort to enable the person to receive necessary treatment. Nevertheless, it is an extraordinary power. Hence the importance of human connection between psychiatrist and patient that transcends a discussion of symptoms of illness and medication.

'I'd like to read you something,' I say to Martin.

He nods.

'This is the weaving of human living: of whose fabric each individual is a part, and of all parts of this fabric, each is intimately connected with the bottom and the extremest reach of time, each is composed of substances identical with the substance of all that surrounds, both the common objects of our disregard, and the hot centres of the stars. James Agee, New York, 1941.' My hands shake, holding the book. Eyes, tears. Unsheathed.

'Very nice,' Martin says. 'How much lithium are you taking?'

'500 mg morning and night. As prescribed. Sir.'

'Any symptoms of psychosis?' he asks.

'No.' I smile.

He doesn't smile back. On his bookshelf are six volumes of Sigmund Freud and various psychiatric texts on mood disorders, anxiety, addictions, relationships and therapy.

'I haven't decided yet, exactly where you fit in the way of diagnosis,' he says.

'In my humble opinion, the brain is way more complex than your international classifications and diagnostic manuals. Have you read this?' I hold up a copy of Toni Morrison's *Beloved*.

'No,' he says.

I sigh. 'It's only one of the best psychological studies of family relationships ever written, never mind the cultural context. All the souls of the world are in here.' I give him my eyes again but he turns away.

'See you in a month,' he says, walking to the door.

Within the month I develop akathisia – a feeling of inner restlessness, an intense compulsion to move, walking or pacing or rocking from one foot to the other. I can't sit down without continually crossing and uncrossing my legs and I can't grip a pen or write a sentence or hold a coffee cup because of the associated tremor in my hands and arms. The exact cause of akathisia is unknown, but it is associated with the older anti-psychotics like pericyazine.

There are other, more serious side effects of these drugs. Muscle rigidity and slowness of movement are common. Tardive dyskinesia can be mistaken for cerebral palsy or spasticity or intellectual disability. It occurs most often in older people who are on long-term therapy. It's a syndrome of involuntary movements: protrusion of the tongue, puffing of the cheeks, puckering of the mouth and chewing. Tardive dyskinesia is usually persistent and irreversible and there is no known treatment.

So Martin suggests seroquel – one of the atypical anti-psychotics now known to be effective for people living with schizophrenia and bipolar mood disorder. To my relief, the transition from one drug to the other is uneventful. The akathisia resolves and the only side effects from the seroquel are dizziness and morning drowsiness. To get out of bed on time for work, I set three different alarms in three different rooms.

Leonardo da Vinci said, 'Painting declines when aloof from nature.' I wonder if wellbeing and spirit do too, and so to find some space and time in which to think, I pack the tent and sleeping bag and food for a week and take some leave from work and drive to the Mt Buffalo National Park. Mt Buffalo is alpine country: pink granite, montane forests, woodland, grassy plains and sphagnum moss in bogs. Bushfires roared through last year and skeletonised most of the snow gums; their once beautiful branches are white and cold. Though everything above ground died, the tree roots survived, and new leaves are feathering up the trunks and lower branches – leaves with blue veins and burnt umber seedpods hanging pendulous as breasts, their tiny black seeds shine like patent leather in the sun.

Out on Wild Dog Plain tors and garlands of granite worn by ice and snow and rain open out into meadows of purple and white flowers. The wind breathes through the tall alpine grass shh shh and as it passes my ears, it sounds a little like arterial blood.

Sex is abundant here. Down low in the undergrowth are paired crickets, beetles and ants, sleek lizards and even the abandoned exoskeletons of cicadas, translucent in the sun. Caterpillars are piled one upon another, devouring leaves. I walk with my mouth slightly open, grinning, and swallow a fly, eeee in the back of my throat. Full-bodied dragonflies flit-start-hover over Dickson's Creek, whose water is here weighed down with algae, further on clear as air. Under the shade of a regenerating snow gum I crouch to the level of everlasting daisies, some great white puffballs of seeds – white parachutes.

The first night is perfect.

The second night is perfect.

The third evening long shadows embrace the grass, swooping through trees, sucking the green. Shadows etch themselves into the ochre pitch of leaves, lengthening into vermilion, blazing against arc cold. My fingers glisten and swerve in leaf-light. I'm cold too. I try wrapping myself around a salmon gum to touch its heat and to kiss its lips as one who is deaf and loving. We glimmer fantastically.

The fourth night the Wandjina come – Kimberley country cloud and rain spirits. Somehow they sneak under my eyelids and even when my eyes are closed, they're . . . staring. They never blink. I sit in the car and listen to the BBC World Service and accidentally catch my reflection in the rearview mirror. Then I'm in the mirror, looking out of the mirror at my reflection. I pack up food and clothes and tent and drive home through the night and in the morning I make an appointment with Martin.

'So,' he says. 'How are you?'

'Oh, a bit weird, intense weird. Very intense weird.'

'What's happening?'

'I've been having visions of spirit people.'

Martin raises his eyebrows. 'Spirit people,' he says.

'Yes. They have black staring eyes or red staring eyes and noses but no mouths. There's a particular Aboriginal name for them but I'm not going to say it out of respect.'

'How many hours of sleep are you getting?'

'Four or five. Depends on what's going on in the night.'

'What's going on in the night?'

'Night-terrors. Nightmares. So I'm teaching myself about surrealism, you know, in art and photography and dream theory and psychology. It's complex, the unconscious and the subconscious – I'm learning instead of sleeping.'

'How's work?'

'What?'

'Work.'

'Oh. Not much in the way of surrealism.'

'Are you still on 300 mg of venlafaxine?'

'Yep.'

'I'd like to reduce the dose.'

'D'you think? I don't know. Intensity of feeling isn't necessarily pathological. Ecstasy may be . . . then again, isn't religious ecstasy considered a higher state of being? Communion with God and enlightenment and all that? If you were a Sufi teacher instead of a psychiatrist, you'd be, I don't know . . . delighted that I'm reaching out to a kind of divine presence.'

Martin leans back in his chair and clasps his hands and looks at me levelly.

'You make things difficult,' he says.

I tense, tense . . . then slacken and sigh and say, 'Okay, what dose?'

'150 mg for a week and we'll review.'

The major mental illnesses – schizophrenia, bipolar disorder and major depression – are biological illnesses. The symptoms result from neurochemical imbalances in the brain. The cause of the neurochemical imbalances is multifactorial: genetics, brain structure, personality, social environment, vulnerability to stress.

Antipsychotic medication, taken consistently, reduces the risk of relapse in individuals with psychosis from 70 per cent to 30 per cent. Antidepressants reduce the risk of depressive relapse by about two thirds. There is a link between psychosocial adversity (major life events and day-to-day difficulties) and illness relapse, but adversity and stress are not sole causal factors. The same applies for use of alcohol and drugs like marijuana and amphetamines.

So, even if we do everything 'right,' if we take our medication, work on cognitive change and behaviour change in therapy, if we manage stress and live reasonably healthily, we still have about a 30 per cent chance of relapse into acute illness.

And sometimes it is hard to identify the early warning signs of relapse, particularly those of hypomania because they're commonly pleasurable – the buzz, the rush of sensory inputs, the energy and euphoria. Sometimes it's like being swept out to sea when you're swept incrementally further out with each wave and you only become aware of how far out you are when you're dangerously distant from the shore.

Martin's office to home is a two-hour walk. Perfect for mulling things over, for reflection. Am I ill? Am I am I . . . I am? Fuck no. No way. Possibly.

'Right,' I say to self. 'Slow down. Think. Deal. What matters?'

There are multi-dimensional consequences of a major relapse – for me and for the people I love and for the people I work with and for the wider community (the costs of hospitalisation). At our regular Saturday night dinner, I say to Zoë and Naava, 'Can I flag something with you?'

'Sure,' they say.

'The thing is . . . for no particular reason . . . everything is kinda intense weird . . . as if god has turned up sound and saturation and contrast. And the nightmares are back. A lot of blood. I think I've been talking too fast. Last night I was trying to explain to Deborah how some numbers are beautiful, like 8, and others are awkward, like 7, and others are mournful, like 9. She really didn't get it. Is that weird?'

'Your theory, or that she didn't understand it?'

'Both.'

'The theory is weird,' says Zoë. 'I don't understand it either.'

'Sure?'

Zoë slides an arm around my shoulders. 'Sorry dude.'

'Damn. Fuck. Blast.'

'Have you been buying stuff?' she asks, gesturing at the pile of new books on the windowsill.

I have to stop and think. 'Possibly.'

'A lot?'

There's an unopened bank statement on the kitchen bench. I open it. Damn.

'It's okay. Do you want to give me your credit card?'

I throw my head back and hit the back of the couch. Groan.

'What are you going to do?' Naava asks.

'I'll go see Jenny next week.'

'Tomorrow,' says Naava. 'I'll come with you.'

'Card please,' says Zoë, holding out her hand gently.

My mum rings later. We talk about their new native garden and about the lamentable state of politics and about the latest shows on TV. I resist the desire to ramble on without pausing and am careful to sound as normal as can be. We're about to hang up and I think I've done pretty well. Then my mum says, 'Are you sure you're okay?'

I say, 'Why?'

'I think you're high. I can hear it in your voice. I've been feeling uneasy all week about you without knowing why.'

'I'm sorry.'

'I'm not asking you to be sorry. I just need to know if you're okay or not.'

I explain about going to see Jenny with Naava.

She sighs. 'We worry so much when you don't tell us what's going on.'

'I keep hoping I'll be back to normal before you have to find out.'

'And then we get a call out of the blue from the hospital.'

Ah. This is clear and present truth.

'You're right,' I say. 'I'm sorry. I'm so sorry. It's because it's a disease of thinking. I think I'm doing the right thing. But I'm not.'

Adequate sleep is essential for moderating mood. Insomnia is known to precipitate and worsen hypomania. Jenny and I decide to increase the seroquel by 100 mg at night and add a very low dose in the day to settle the racing thoughts and agitation. It's true that small dose increases early on (at night if possible to reduce side effects) can circumvent the later need for large dose increases. We talk about reframing odd thoughts and not catastrophising, or automatically assuming things will get worse.

'Let's catch up in a few days,' Jenny says. 'In the meantime, you know what to do.'

So here I am, a mentally ill patient participating in the management of my own illness. Given clear and honest information about treatments, I think most of us do want to have an active voice in decision-making (when we're able).

On the weekends I go walking in the Brisbane Ranges National Park for physical exercise, wilderness, trees, air, the vast expansion of sky and perspective. I take medication as directed. To manage the fleeting auditory hallucinations and the sudden erratic ideas, I reply (in thought) with 'Does that make sense?' or 'Is this the most likely explanation?' or 'That's ridiculous,' or 'Oh, piss off.'

At work I observe others' body language. If they're frowning or looking confused or bored, I try to rein in the train of thought and shut-up. If someone I trust says, 'You're not making sense,' they're almost certainly right – I'm not making sense.

It takes a couple of weeks. It's hard walking along the precipice. Sometimes I waver. Then the sustained absence of symptoms brings relief, like the absence of physical pain after a period of suffering. The bank balance is battered, but otherwise I'm okay.

Martin's waiting room is dusky pink and somehow its physical presence and its pinkness are a visceral reminder of being unwell. I sit uneasily here and hold tight to my pile of books.

Martin comes out of his office as he always does – stiffly.

'Hi Sarah,' he says.

I look to see if anyone else is in the room and then stand up.

'Kate,' I say, tapping my sternum.

'Oh,' he says.

We wade through the standard set of psychiatric questions to be found in any standard medical textbook. Neither of us is particularly interested in either the questions or the answers. The feel in the room is flat as concrete. After eight minutes he ushers me out and I pay the bill and walk down the stairs and take a tram to the beach. Solace is right here – sitting on a pier in the sun, listening to water suckling rocks near the shore.

Then I walk back towards the city and pass a hair salon. There is nothing special about this particular salon, except that I'm passing it in a brave mood. For years I've cut my hair with the kitchen scissors. I go inside to see what might happen.

The salon apprentice is about seventeen. Skinny. Tight-jeanned. His lips are pink with just the hint of gloss-shine. He asks me to lean right back in the chair in front of a basin and he scoops up my hair from the base of my skull and turns on the water. Little electric currents run across my head, down my arms and spine. He rubs shampoo through my hair. It smells like orange blossom. The electric currents find the tips of my toes. Now I can't feel my legs. I'm floating. His fingers are like warm water, like molasses, like . . . oh, the touch of another human being. I want to run away and I want to give in to it. He slows down and presses in, gently, and I give in to it.

31

'There's a continuum,' Winsome says the following week, 'for all of us in our adult lives, from emptiness to meaning. And meaning . . . meaning comes from family, relationships, spirituality, work . . . you know this stuff, it's not quantum mechanics.'

'Yes,' I say. 'We all want to be loved. We all want to feel connected. It doesn't have to be to someone – it could be to something.' I shuffle in the chair. 'That's where I think mental illness really sucks. It makes it harder to feel loved and it can make it much harder to give love.'

'There's another continuum: from chaos to control, in your living circumstances and relationships, finances and health. When you first came to see me–'

'Chaos,' I say.

'Yes. And now?'

'I know what I need to do to stay well . . . as well as I can.'

'And?'

'I think . . . if I'm able to control this illness instead of it controlling me, then rather than lurching from one crisis to the next . . . I'm free to manage the present better. You know, to be able to plan stuff, even simple stuff like having friends over for dinner – that's a big thing. For so many years I couldn't do that because there was no guarantee of a sound mind from one week to the next.'

'What else?'

'Now there's the possibility of a future.'

'Indeed. Just keep going,' Winsome says.

So I do. I do, I will. This isn't my second chance, this is my sixteenth chance. How many people are lucky enough to get a sixteenth chance?

So.

So what is the essence? What matters . . . what really, really matters . . . is it giving love? Is it procreation? Is it knowledge, is it finding truth? The struggle to overcome, relief from pain? Is it stillness? The scraps of nirvana? Perhaps it's connection. Visceral connection and part of the journey together and touching souls. We.

My last day on earth may be cloudy. Or the sun may blaze. At the moment of my last breath someone will be born. Someone will discover the poetry of W.H. Auden. Someone will see a bird in the sky for the very first time. Someone will forget milk for the morning coffee.

Nietzsche writes, 'Life consists of rare, isolated moments of the greatest significance, and of innumerably many intervals, during which at best the silhouettes of those moments hover about us.'

Yes.

He continues, 'Love, springtime, every beautiful melody, mountains, the moon, the sea—all these speak completely to the heart but once, if in fact they ever do get a chance to speak completely.'

Oh no. No. Every time I go to a live gig and the background music finally sighs out and the lights dim there's that moment of blackness and silence in which I forget to breathe until the first guitar note of the first song when my heart rushes right out of my chest and gives itself, all of its red beating self, to the musicians and their music. And tonight, an ordinary Friday night, I'm sitting here on the couch that the cats use as a scratching post, alone with the precious things of the night. Music in the night. Bach's Suite for Solo Cello no. 2 in D Minor. One soul (the composer's) communing with another (the player's) communing with another (the listener's) – alighting together at the same place and point in the universe, an exact moment, thrilling and pure: some might call it divine.

32

In the same way people with severe allergies carry an EpiPen, I now carry a supply of low dose, emergency medication, and I take it whenever a vague sense of paranoia creeps up or when something ordinary takes on undue meaning. For a full 24 hours in every 12–14 days I learn to deliberately reduce all forms of stimulation and withdraw to one room for sleep, solitude and silence. Healing time. Regenerating time. Recalibrating time. It seems that in conjunction with medication, the brain requires a period of stillness in which to re-establish equilibrium. Any fleeting symptoms of illness dissipate. I re-enter the world a 'relatively normal' person.

As often as possible I pack the tent and a bag of provisions. The road to Mt Buffalo at dawn is a theatre of mist, of ghosts rising and contorting and falling away. The mist clears near the plateau; up the steep track to Corral Peak is a lone granite tor, Sentinel, reaching right into the blue of the sky. Kookaburras note my slow approach – five of them at least – laughing in stereo to the north and south and east and west. All the hairs are up on my legs and arms and I shiver, then laugh, then cry.

Now the echo of crows on the cliff face.

The highest point of the National Park is called The Horn and from here I can see across to the Bogong High Plains and Mt Beauty. I walk down from the summit, off the track, in between the snow gums and unwittingly fall asleep on a soft mound which turns out to be an ants' nest and when I wake some hours later I'm covered in shiny red ants and the sun is cradled between two branches, one above one below, both in shadow, paying homage.

Day-smell is different from dusk-smell is different from night-smell. Day-smell is warmed eucalyptus oil and mountain tea-tree, candle heath and aromatic alpine baekea. Dusk-smell is thick with native grasses and boronia. Night-smell is the deep cool water of Lake Catani, where the other-side sun is reflecting onto the moon and the moon dribbles light over the still water of the lake and I open my body to it, skin white as the moon.

Flesh, air. A breathing silence.

Meaning. Illness. This thing called life.

Currawongs are the first sound of the morning, followed by flies around the entrance to my tent and the deeper sound of bees. I crawl outside to find a flame robin in a near-by eucalypt. He takes flight. I walk down to the lake for a swim, for the water like silk and the bottom-silt like silk. In front of me, as I glide along, are two wood ducks and the occasional plop! and ripple of a fish. Bright-eyed butterflies, brown and orange like a checkerboard, flicker together just above the surface. On the other side of the lake I look for frogs and cicadas in the alpine bog, but they grow faint and vow silence whenever I come close. So I sit and wait.

By my wet feet is a grass trigger plant with magenta flowers on a long single stalk that turn to slender blood-red seeds at the very top. Then a sudden, low flrrrr –birds' wings – quite close, I swing around . . . the wind is whispering the leaves and weathered silver branches of the mountain gums.

Back at my tent I eat some fruit and take the lithium and seroquel and venlafaxine with water and then I write for a while – playing around with words till they start to sing. I pack my backpack and walk – out towards the west edge of the plateau, walk till my calves and thighs are stretched and quietly sore. In the early evening I ease down into the grass and heath, disturbing some grasshoppers, rather ripe-looking and violent green.

In the sky are long streaks of cloud.

Why do I look at a group of yellowgold daisies and lose my breath? Is it that they remind me of the sun? Why do I know they are perfect? I'm not a bee or a bird; I can't pollinate them. Perhaps it's the symmetry or perhaps it's evolutionary. Perhaps it has something to do with Jung's collective unconscious or is it merely their contrast with the pale alpine grass? The daisies have soft yellow centres with an orange rim. Then the yellowgold petals – six of them, darkest gold at the base, brightest yellow nearest the floret. They couldn't possibly be more alive. When I sit up, my abdomen is mired with wombat shit. I wonder if wombats ever go mad or if insanity is peculiarly human.

I take off my boots and thick socks and feel the native grass under my feet. It is surprisingly soft. I take off my glasses and listen to the dusk. To my right a kookaburra, rrrlaaah hah hahhah haw, to my left tiny yellow-faced honeyeaters are settling in for the night. They are no bigger than my thumb. They zip from tree to tree, hee ee ee. Crimson rosellas call to one another across the valley. How quickly I'm surrounded by the zing of fat march flies. Why do they bother with me? Is it the warmth of my body? Perhaps as I lie amongst the alpine grass and snow gums they are waiting for the softness of dead flesh in which to lay their larvae. Their wings flutter over my eyelids. I'm waiting for wombats to come up out of their holes into the dusk.

I listen and wait. Ah, the moon behind a strand of eucalypts. Moths, dark and flittering against the paler sky.

Once the sun has dipped below the mountain range the march flies leave and the mosquitoes come and the moon rises behind a stand of eucalypts. The smell of dusk air. The moon is each minute brighter. The birds are all quiet now – just the sound of frogs and cicadas and forest bats overhead and the wind shhh through the tops of the trees. Then the kookaburra again rrlaah hah hah haw. Now the stars. First one, then another then another. Blinking, as they do. Then the frogs and cicadas stop, then no wind.

So quiet. Still. A million stars.

Mental illness happens to people who are living ordinary, good lives, just like my family and me when I first became ill. And for the families, friends and carers of people with mental illness it is particularly hard because the illness can take away our ability to know that we are loved, and we often find it hard to love back in conventional ways. For some of us, after a while we forget how to love.

For me, staying well is a daily job of monitoring mood and thinking and keeping regular rhythms of waking and sleeping. I take medication every morning and evening, and will do so for all of my life. At thirty-eight, I've been well for around four years but I'm not 'cured'. Good health doesn't come with a guarantee for anyone, but for those of us managing a long-term illness, each day of wellness is, in its own small way, remarkable.

I'm grateful to be living in a country where medication and therapy are mostly available and affordable. However even in Australia, we are still not caring for the most vulnerable members of our communities. Those who, through no fault of their own, are not as lucky as I have been to respond to medication or to be able to afford to find the right kind of therapy. These people are of all ages and backgrounds, and we ignore their suffering because most of us don't understand their ways of seeing the world or we are afraid of their difference or embarrassed by their appearance and because we can't see their injuries.

No-one ever wakes up one morning and thinks, today I'd like to go mad, lose my job and friends, and end up odd-looking and living on the streets, *anymore than they think,* today I'd like to get cancer.

AFTERWORD

By Winsome Thomas

Kate Richards is one of the most courageous and intelligent clients I have ever had the opportunity to work with.

Kate's first session took place on 19 April 2004. She came without referral having just seen my brochure at street level. When asked how I could help her she said that she had suffered episodes of depression since the age of fifteen and had been hospitalised for electroconvulsive therapy (ECT). She had been on medication for about ten years and was taking a mood stabiliser and an antidepressant. Two months prior she had deliberately burned herself with hydrochloric acid. That session marked the commencement of our five-year journey.

All therapy is an excursion into the behaviours, emotions, life and mind of the client. Some relationships are intense and some are gentle. All relationships endure only while the client has issues. Most last several sessions but Kate's relationship with me was much longer. It covered considerable periods when she was hospitalised (usually after a suicide attempt or a psychotic episode) and then later resumed therapy after several weeks. Her illness was much more severe than most. Here was a young woman who suffered from a mental illness that failed to have a definitive diagnosis – not that the label per se would have assisted a great deal. It was sufficient to say that she was very ill and that her symptoms indicated the presence of psychosis and major depression.

I recall two major turning points in her therapy.

The first occurred early on when Kate spent quite some time during the session walking up and down in the room and avoiding real engagement. I challenged her and said something like, 'Kate, you can entertain me for as long as you like but it will not help you. I'm not playing games here.' She sat down, looked at me very seriously and later said that I was the first therapist that she had been able to trust.

The second took place much later. Conformity with desired doses of medication was a real issue for Kate. She had trained as a doctor and knew a great deal about drugs, their effects and which ones suited her or not. It was she who discovered that a relatively 'old' medication alleviated her nightmares. At each session I would ask her about her symptoms, her lifestyle (for example her diet, sleep patterns, supports, work and use of alcohol) and her compliance with the medication prescribed. At times Kate would either not take her medication or would adjust it in a way that she thought appropriate without blood samples having been taken. Of course, her stability fluctuated accordingly.

One day in a session I said to Kate something like, 'You know Kate, you have a mental illness. Once you admit that and acknowledge that you cannot live without your medication then your life will change.' I recall the long pause that ensued with Kate looking at me and then shifting her gaze while squirming in her seat. She finally acknowledged the truth of my statement. That was the turning point. Thereafter she started to take her medication appropriately.

In my view, therapy is both an art and a science. Intuition, relationship and trust are essential components. Throughout therapy I called a spade a spade and did not resile from discussions about suicide plans. As a result the knife in the kitchen drawer was to be brought to the next session or was to be put well away from reach. Kate suggested the roof. If she were to become psychotic she was to phone me and/or friends and/or family. Names and numbers were to be accessible. Much discussion took place about doctors, hospitals, medication and psychiatrists. We talked about who could she trust, what meds were appropriate for her and where she felt safe. Each was a major hurdle in itself.

Later, our slow journey focused on normalising her life. Here's a sample:

'No, ten espresso coffees do not constitute an appropriate diet.'

'It's ok for someone to touch and hug you.'

'No, you can't stay up all night, a regular sleep pattern is required.'

'Supermarkets are not places to be feared and haunted at 11.00 p.m. at night.'

We also talked about prosaic issues such as buying underwear or clothes that fitted, wearing makeup, taking a bath and relationships with others. We determined what was essential in a basic life and lifestyle and what were optional extras. I felt immense compassion for this young woman who struggled with the very basics of life.

My work with Kate, as it is with each client, was forensic, cognitive and analytical – not to mention, immensely challenging and thoroughly rewarding. I never had any doubts regarding Kate's intelligence. I'm now so pleased that I encouraged her to return to her passion for writing and to enrol in the writing course at RMIT. This book is a testament to her great skill, tenacity and insight.

Kate's journey has been painful indeed in so many ways. Her capacity to endure, to reflect, to trust and to survive is remarkable. How privileged I have been to walk the journey of recovery with her.

20 November 2012

ACKNOWLEDGEMENTS

To my parents, Cliff and Norma Richards.

To Zoë and Naava – without whom I wouldn't be here.

To my soul mate Dr Peh Tan Ying.

To Karen Manton for teaching me to write and revere.

To Winsome Thomas (MAPS) for finding a path and making the journey safe.

To Tanya Ramm, Sarah Clark, Dr Melyse Hearne, Dr Lara Verplak and Deborah Cruickshank for the years of friendship that continue to mean so much.

To 'Anna' (RN), 'Damien' (RN) and the many other mental health nurses who demonstrate that compassion and innovation and hope are alive in the public mental health system.

To Dr Jenny Jobst (FRACGP), 'Helen' (MAPS), Monica Manton (MAPS) and Dr Sophie Richmond (FRACGP) for *listening*, and for always taking mental health and mental illness seriously.

To wonderful fellow writers for their keen insight, generosity and support and for all the evenings of illumination (and wine): Dr Susan Gardiner, Dana Miltins, Trish Bolton, Jenny Green, Lucy Treolar, Susan Biggar, Carolyn Ingvarson, Helen Rushford, Greg Foyster, Jill Stansfield, Julie Twohig, Harry Blutstein, Heather Rose.

To RMIT Professional Writing and Editing teachers-mentors-friends: Di Websdale-Morrissey, Toni Jordan, Malcolm King, Dr Olga Lorenzo.

To Jane Matthews, Christine Russell, Rachel Koelmeyer, Joanne Dean, Monique Anderson and Bev McClure at PMCC.

To Lyn Batchelor, Win and Alex Fox, Adele Green, Tori Smith, Alain Behar, Judith Fleming and Sharyn Moloney.

To the team at Monash Alfred Psychiatry Research Centre (MAPrc) – 'mending minds' through clinical research.

To Andrea McNamara at Penguin for believing in the possibility, and for breaking in a rather barbarous manuscript with such grace.

WHERE TO GO FOR HELP

MENTAL HEALTH INFORMATION AND SUPPORT

Mental Illness Fellowship of Australia

National helpline: 1800 985 944

www.mifa.org.au

Mental Health Associations/Foundations

Information, research, programs, services and links:

NSW:	1300 794 991	www.mentalhealth.asn.au
NT:	1300 780 081	www.teamhealth.asn.au
SA:	(08) 8378 4100	www.mifa.org.au/mifsa
QLD:	1300 729 686	www.mentalhealth.org.au
VIC:	(03) 9826 1422	www.mentalhealthvic.org.au
WA:	(08) 9420 7277	www.waamh.org.au
TAS:	1800 332 388 (Mental Health Helpline)	

Mi Networks peer support line

Australia-wide support, information and referral to local services:

1800 985 944

SANE Australia

A national charity working for a better life for people affected by mental illness:

SANE Helpline: 1800 187 263

www.sane.org

Beyond Blue

The national depression initiative

Information Line: 1300 22 4636

www.beyondblue.org.au

Mental Health Carers Arafmi Australia (MHCAA)

http://www.arafmiaustralia.asn.au/

National e-mental health online portal

http://www.mindhealthconnect.org.au/

CRISIS SUPPORT SERVICES

Public Emergency Mental Health Services

For 24-hour local contact numbers, contact the hospitals in your area, or check the White Pages under 'Mental Health' or look up State Government websites.

The Suicide Call Back Service

Crisis counselling 24 hours per day 7 days a week across Australia.

1300 659 467

www.suicidecallbackservice.org.au/

Lifeline
    13 11 14
    www.lifeline.org.au

Kids Help Line
    1800 55 1800
    www.kidshelpline.com.au

Ambulance, Police, Fire
    000